# Understanding Dental Health

# Understanding Dental Health

**Francis G. Serio, D.M.D., M.S.**

*Understanding Health and Sickness Series, Miriam Bloom, Editor*
University Press of Mississippi
Jackson

01  00  99  98    4  3  2  1
The paper in this book meets the guidelines for permanence and durability
of the Committee on Production Guidelines for Book Longevity of the
Council on Library Resources.

Illustrations by Regan Causey Tuder

Library of Congress Cataloging-in-Publication Data

Serio, Francis G.
        Understanding dental health / Francis G. Serio.
            p.    cm.—(Understanding health and sickness series)
        Includes bibliographical references and index.
        ISBN 1-57806-009-5 (cloth : alk. paper).—ISBN 1-57806-010-9
(paper : alk. paper)
        1. Dentistry—Popular works.    2. Teeth—Care and hygiene.
I. Title.    II. Series.
RK61.S47    1998
617.6—dc21                                                    97-15276
                                                                CIP

British Library Cataloging-in-Publication data available

# Contents

## Acknowledgments and Dedication

I would like to thank Dr. Miriam Bloom, general editor of the Understanding Health and Sickness Series at the University Press of Mississippi, for her guidance and support and Dr. Howard E. Strassler of the University of Maryland Dental School for reviewing the manuscript. I am especially grateful to Dr. Cheryl L. Serio, my own dentist and my best friend, for allowing me to pursue my professional and personal dreams.

This book is dedicated to my father, the late Joseph Serio, D.D.S., who taught me to love dentistry as a profession.

# Introduction

Looking into your mouth is in some ways like looking under the hood of your car. Both are dark and mysterious places, each having its own particular aroma, and you generally have little idea what you are looking at. You would like to know more, and for your car you would get out the owner's manual and read it. But what about for your mouth? Unfortunately, your mouth did not come with an owner's manual; you have only the information your mother, your dentist, and some semienlightened writers have given you. Both your car and your mouth will run better with a bit of preventive maintenance. Changing the oil in your engine will give you a greater chance of additional years of trouble-free service; so will removing the plaque from your teeth. This book is designed to provide you with information that will help you understand your mouth and how to keep it in good shape.

The mouth is one of the most important parts of the human body. It serves a survival function as the portal of entry and initial processing point for food. It allows you to speak, which is the primary mode of communication in your daily life. Strong emotions, positive and negative, are transmitted both through spoken words and through the shapes formed by the mouth and lips.

Your mouth contributes greatly to your overall appearance and sense of self. A bright, cheery smile with a display of beautiful "white" teeth always gets a positive response. It is one of your most important nonverbal cues when you see someone, whether it's for the first or the thousandth time. Cosmetic and toothpaste companies spend, and make, fortunes marketing products intended to create a more pleasing smile.

In contrast, people who are self-conscious about their mouths may not smile at all, may smile with their lips pursed tightly over their teeth, or may cover their mouths with their hands. An unsightly smile detracts from an otherwise attractive appearance.

Although clothes may "make the person," a pleasant smile completes the ensemble.

"Don't take it personally, Doc, but I hate coming to the dentist!" is an all-too-common refrain heard in many dental offices. Sometimes this sentiment is based on previous experience, but often it is culturally engendered. Jokes about the agonies of root canals or gum surgery pervade modern culture. Horror stories about visits to the dentist are traded at beauty salons and over cold beers. Well-meaning parents, when taking children to a first dental appointment, tell them that it's not going to hurt (thus introducing the possibility that it might). In reality, most dental treatment is almost completely painless, or, at worst, is mildly uncomfortable. The advances in modern pain control, including the use of local anesthetics ("novocaine," which is actually usually lidocaine) administered with narrow, razor-sharp needles, nitrous oxide (laughing gas) analgesia, the appropriate use of sedatives, and the pre- and posttreatment use of nonsteroidal anti-inflammatory analgesics have taken most of the pain out of dental treatment. "Painless Parker," a dentist in New York City in the 1920s and 1930s, would feel right at home in modern dentistry.

For many people it is the fear of pain that leads to procrastination in seeking help for dental problems. Dental pain usually has a readily detectable cause. It may be related to decay in a tooth, transient damage to gingival (gum) tissue, an abscess, or a canker sore or other mouth ulcer. If related to a decayed tooth or gum abscess, the pain may pass temporarily but often returns at a higher level. This cycle may continue until the pain is unbearable (usually late on a Saturday night), and damage that is irreversible or that will involve costly treatment has occurred.

The truth is that modern dentistry, especially in the area of prevention, has progressed to the point where, in most cases, caries (decay) and periodontal (gum) disease are preventable. You can maintain your teeth and gums in a healthy and comfortably functioning state for your entire life, though it will require a bit of daily attention on your part. This book, which covers the major aspects of dental care, will help you achieve that goal.

Because of size limitations, some topics are only briefly discussed. Chapter 1 outlines the anatomy of the mouth. Chapter 2 discusses your responsibilities related to daily oral hygiene and maintenance, what your dentist's job is with respect to a complete examination, and some financial aspects (cost and payment) of dental care. Chapter 3 covers dental caries (decay), explaining what it is, how it occurs and can be avoided, and what is involved in the repair or replacing of decayed teeth. Chapter 4 deals with periodontal disease (in actuality a collection of diseases), which affects the teeth's supporting structures in about 95% of the population in one form or another. Chapter 5 covers crooked teeth and orthodontics (braces). Chapter 6 is a discussion of various other oral maladies such as viral infections, oral cancer, "TMJ," and halitosis (bad breath) and includes preventive tips and treatment options. Chapter 7 describes new technology such as lasers, intraoral cameras, video imaging, and computer-assisted design and fabrication of restorations (CAD-CAM). Chapter 8 provides an update on dental research and sheds light on some long-standing controversies in dentistry. For those who would like further information, chapter 9 and the appendices list a variety of sources available through all types of media, including the Internet.

While it would be reassuring to believe that everything done in dentistry has a scientific basis, this is simply not the case. Insofar as it is possible, I will present state-of-the-art conclusions as supported by current literature. Occasionally, my own opinion will hold sway, and I will try to make it clear when this is the case.

# Understanding Dental Health

# 1. The Mouth

As you read this chapter, you may want to have a mirror handy so that you can examine the various parts of your own mouth, as shown in figure I–I.

## TISSUES

The mouth comprises a variety of tissues. There are six major tissue types which contribute in various forms to the structure of the mouth. The epithelium acts as the covering for all of the soft tissues. The connective tissue, with its collection of fibers, blood vessels and nerves, is found under the epithelium. The epithelium and connective tissue act as the covering for the jawbones, as well as for the other bones in your body. The teeth are made from enamel (the structure most often visible), dentin, which constitutes the bulk of the tooth, and cementum, which covers the surface of the root.

The epithelium—the tissue that covers and protects the entire body, including the inside of the mouth—has different structures and functions depending on its location. In the mouth, the epithelium serves as the covering for the cheeks, lips, gingiva (gums), tongue, and other soft tissue surfaces. A specialized type of epithelium covers the top of the tongue and gives rise to the taste buds and papillae which give the tongue its unique appearance and function.

The surface of the epithelium may be covered with keratin, the thickened outer coating of protein which gives epithelium its toughness. Epithelium is classified as being either keratinized or unkeratinized. Gingiva, the tissue which surrounds the tooth, is covered with keratinized epithelium. This thickened surface of keratin gives the gingiva its usual light-pink appearance. In many cases, the gingiva is also stippled, giving the tissue a roughened

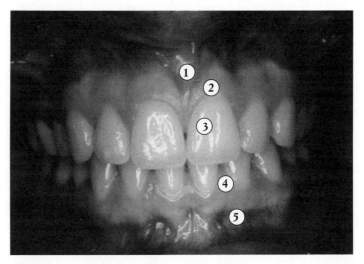

1. Frenum    2. Gingival Margin    3. Tooth Crown
4. Gingiva   5. Alveolar Mlicosa

FIG I–I: Visible anatomy of the mouth

appearance, similar to the skin of an orange. Sometimes the gingiva has a degree of brown pigmentation; though this occurs most often in persons of African descent, it can be found in those with any pigmented skin. Occasionally, Caucasians may also have some lightly pigmented gingiva. The gingiva is firmly bound down to the underlying jawbone and is not moveable.

The tissue next to the gingiva is called the alveolar mucosa. This tissue is covered with nonkeratinized epithelium. The alveolar mucosa is moveable and not bound down to the underlying bone. Because of the thinness of nonkeratinized epithelium, the surface blood vessels in the underlying connective tissue can be seen easily; they give the alveolar mucosa a redder appearance than the gingiva.

The cells which make up the epithelium turn over or change at varying rates, making these cells susceptible to mutational changes, some of which may be harmful. Such changes may be caused by alcohol, tobacco, sunlight, or constant trauma to the tissues. One layer of the epithelium, the basal layer, is quite sensitive to the sun. The recent alarming increase in cases of basal cell carcinoma (skin cancer) of the face is directly related to the exposure of skin that occurs during suntanning. The use of cigarettes and smokeless tobacco has been definitely linked to the occurrence of oral cancer, particularly squamous cell carcinoma, a type of epithelial cancer.

Beneath the epithelium is the connective tissue. This tissue is predominantly collagen (a type of protein) with a variety of protein-sugar complexes. Blood vessels and nerve endings are embedded in the connective tissue. The main functions of connective tissue are to support and hold the body together. In periodontal disease, it is the connective tissue which becomes inflamed and is eventually destroyed. Bone is connective tissue which is calcified or hardened. The same inflammatory processes which attack the connective tissue also attack and destroy bone. Tooth loss due to periodontal disease is directly attributable to this destruction of bone.

## TEETH

Figure 1–2 illustrates the typical anatomy of a tooth, which has three main parts. The crown, which is usually visible in the mouth, is covered with enamel, the hardest substance in the body. Enamel is usually a whitish-to-pale-yellow color. It is also translucent, allowing light to pass through it. The tips of the incisors (teeth will be identified by name below) sometimes look a little grayish because light passes through them and is not stopped by any underlying dentin. The dentin makes up the bulk of the tooth and is normally a shade of yellow. Depending on the shade of dentin and the thickness and shade of enamel, the tooth crown may appear to be more yellow than white. Over time, teeth tend to become stained and yellow as a result of exposure to coffee, tea, wine, cola and other soft drinks, and

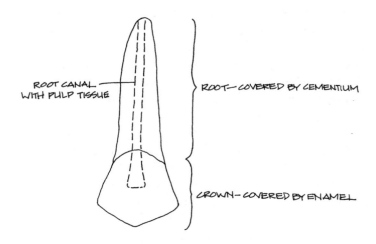

FIG I–2: Anatomy of a tooth

cigarettes. Certain medications can also discolor teeth. Dentin is less mineralized than enamel, which makes it more susceptible to tooth decay (see chapter 3).

The second part is the root, an elongated structure which anchors the tooth in the jaw. The root is composed predominantly of dentin with a thin covering of cementum, specialized hard tooth tissue which helps the root attach to the gingiva and alveolar bone. When a root becomes exposed due to recession of the gingiva, the tooth may become sensitive to cold, hot, or sweets. Exposed roots are also susceptible to decay.

The root of the tooth contains the third major structure, the pulp. The pulp is a collection of connective tissue, blood vessels, and nerves which fill the root canal, a narrow channel in the center of the root. The pulp tissue formed all of the dentin of the tooth during development and still has some dentin-producing capacity. When it becomes infected by dental caries, the pulp may become quite painful or necrose, with resulting infection and further pain. In these instances, endodontic (root canal) therapy is necessary to remove the damaged or dead tissue and preserve the tooth.

When all of the permanent (adult) teeth have erupted, most adults will have 32 teeth. In this respect, the mouth is bilaterally symmetric, with the same types of teeth in the maxillary (upper) arch and the mandibular (lower) arch. Each arch can be divided in half, called quadrants. Each quadrant will have, starting from the middle, a central incisor, lateral incisor, canine (cuspid), first and second premolar (bicuspids), first molar (6-year molar), second molar (12-year molar), and third molar (wisdom tooth). In one arch, each tooth has the same shape on the right and left side. The maxillary teeth and mandibular teeth with corresponding names have somewhat different shapes.

The incisors are designed for biting through food and therefore have sharp edges similar to a shovel's. Incisors also help in the pronunciation of words. The canines, used for tearing, have sharp points at the ends, called cusps. The premolars and molars provide chewing surfaces for the grinding of food. These teeth have both cusps (peaks) and fossas (valleys), with the number and arrangement depending on the particular tooth. The molars also provide support when the teeth are brought together.

Incisors and canines generally have one root. Maxillary first premolars usually have two roots; maxillary second premolars and mandibular premolars usually have one. Maxillary first and second molars usually have three roots, although the second molar roots may be fused together. Mandibular first and second molars have two roots. Both maxillary and mandibular third molars come in a variety of shapes and sizes with no predictable morphologic pattern. Associated with each root is the root canal and pulp. In most instances, there is one canal per root. Occasionally, a second canal may be present. If this smaller canal is not found during root canal therapy, that therapy may not be successful. The general shape of each tooth type is illustrated in figure 1–3.

As humans have evolved, the cranial vault, which houses the brain, has enlarged while the jaws have become smaller. Some people may be missing some, or all, of the third molars. Consider yourself evolutionarily advanced if you are missing some of your

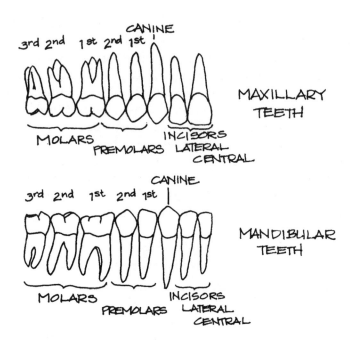

FIG 1–3: Anatomy of each tooth type

wisdom teeth! Occasionally, another tooth, usually a second premolar or maxillary lateral incisor, may also be congenitally missing.

Children have 20 primary (deciduous, baby, milk) teeth. A child will have two central incisors, two lateral incisors, two canines, two first molars, and two second molars in each arch. The primary teeth serve several important functions. They are used, of course, for eating. They also help in the development of the jaws and save space for the eventual arrival of the permanent teeth. The notion that they are "just" baby teeth and hence do not need to be cared for is totally erroneous. Decay in primary teeth can lead to abscesses which damage the permanent successor teeth underneath. The premature loss of primary teeth may adversely affect the eruption of the permanent teeth which will succeed them.

The eruption sequence and timing of both the deciduous and permanent teeth is important to parents and children alike (an interest personified in the tooth fairy). The mandibular primary central and lateral incisors are the first to erupt, when a child is about 6–7 months of age. The maxillary central and lateral incisors follow shortly thereafter. The first molars arrive at 12–14 months, followed by the mandibular and maxillary canines at 16–18 months. The set of primary teeth is completed by the 24th month with the arrival of the second molars.

In the permanent dentition, the sequence of eruption of the maxillary teeth starts with the first molars (6-year molar), followed by the central incisors, lateral incisors, first premolars, second premolars, canines, and second molars (12-year molars). The eruption sequence is generally finished in the early teen years. The third molars will erupt, if they do so at all, in the late teen years into the early twenties. The mandibular sequence of eruption is similar to the canines erupting after the lateral incisors, then the first and second premolars, with the second molars bringing up the rear. In actuality, there is wide variance in the timing of eruption from one child to another, even among siblings. If you have a concern about delayed eruption, your dentist can make a radiograph (X-ray film) to show which of your child's teeth are present under the gums.

## JAWBONES

Underneath the connective tissue of the gingiva and alveolar mucosa into which the teeth are embedded are the jawbones. The maxilla is the upper jawbone, and the mandible is the lower one. The teeth are anchored in the alveolar process of the jaws by their roots and are connected to the bone by the periodontal ligament (PDL). This relationship is demonstrated in figure 1–4. The PDL is a type of connective tissue that helps to protect the teeth by absorbing the shock of chewing and of the teeth coming together. The PDL also contains a nerve reflex arc which allows

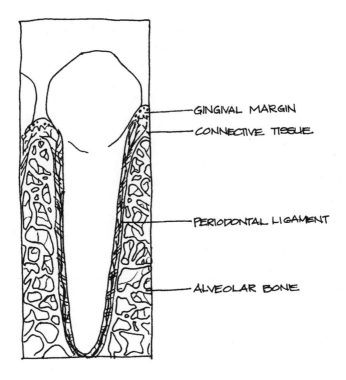

FIG I–4: The relationship of a tooth to the gingiva and alveolar bone

the mandible to open automatically when someone encounters a hard object while chewing (such as bone in a piece of meat). It is important to note that it is the mandible which moves during chewing and speaking. When the dentist asks you to bite down, you are really biting up (if you were asked to bite up, you would have no idea what to do).

If teeth are lost due to caries or periodontal disease, the jawbone which held the missing teeth will begin to deteriorate. In extreme circumstances, all of the alveolar process is lost, with only the basal bone of the maxilla and mandible remaining. In these situations, it is almost impossible to wear a complete denture. The weakened mandible is also susceptible to fracture from even very mild forces. It is the alveolar process which is also destroyed by periodontitis, the type of periodontal disease which attacks the tooth-supporting bone.

## SALIVARY GLANDS AND TONGUE

The alveolar mucosa leads to the vestibule of the mouth, which then connects to the buccal mucosa, or cheek. The buccal mucosa is also lined with nonkeratinized epithelium. Because it has fewer blood vessels and some underlying muscle and fat, the buccal mucosa may not appear as red as the alveolar mucosa. The buccal mucosa also has many minor salivary and mucous glands embedded within it. These glands can often be felt as little bumps with your tongue, especially near the lips.

The mouth also contains several major salivary glands. The sublingual and submandibular glands empty their contents under the tongue. These glands account for the pooling of saliva in this area. The saliva, particularly from the submandibular gland with its content of calcium and phosphate, contributes to the formation of dental calculus (tartar) on the lingual (tongue side) surface of the mandibular incisors. The other major salivary glands are the parotid glands, located in the cheeks. If you have had the mumps, you are familiar with these glands. The parotid glands empty through ducts next to the maxillary first molars, which you can feel as a bump on the inside of your cheek with your tongue. Your saliva contains enzymes which begin to digest your food even while you are still chewing. The saliva helps control the pH, or acidity, in your mouth. The lubricating and lavage action of the saliva is important in chewing, swallowing, and cleansing of the mouth.

The other major visible structure of the mouth is your tongue. The dorsal (top) surface of the tongue is covered with specialized epithelium. The bulk of the dorsum of the tongue is covered by thin filiform papillae and mushroom-like fungiform papillae with associated taste buds. More taste buds are located in the posterior one-third of the tongue with the circumvallate papillae. Foliate papillae are found on the lateral borders of the tongue. In humans, the filiform papillae are quite soft and prone to staining, especially in conjunction with cigarette smoking. In cats, the filiform papillae are rough to aid in cleansing the fur.

You may have noticed that certain parts of your tongue are sensitive to different flavors. The four basic categories of taste are sweet, salt, sour, and bitter; taste buds for each of these are distributed regionally. Taste buds for sweet and salt are found in the anterior to middle third of the tongue, those for sour in the middle and back, and those for bitter in the back. Take a pinch of salt or sugar and notice where you "feel" the taste.

## FACIAL MUSCLES

Surrounding the mouth and embedded within the cheeks and face are the muscle groups which allow the face and mouth to function. These are divided into two main groups: muscles of facial expression and muscles of mastication. The muscles of facial expression change the shape of the face and lips. A person with the condition known as Bell's palsy will have paralysis of some of the muscles of facial expression. The result is that one side of the face sags due to the loss of muscle tonicity. Occasionally, these muscles are also affected by local anesthetics, which may cause the same kind of droopy appearance. As alarming as this may be initially, the muscles return to their normal shape and function as the anesthetic wears off.

The muscles of mastication allow the mandible to open and close and also balance the mandible when biting force is being generated. The mandible is attached to the rest of the skull by a hinge, the temporomandibular joint (TMJ). This joint is held together by ligaments and muscles. There is a disc of cartilage, the meniscus, which is located between the end of the mandible, or condyle, and the fossa in which the condyle sits. Patients who have TMJ trouble may have problems with the muscles of mastication or with the joint itself (see chapter 6).

# 2. An Ounce of Prevention: What You and Your Dentist Can Do

## YOUR JOB

In this day and age, most common dental problems are completely preventable. Of course, there is no such thing as a free lunch. Good oral health results from daily attention to proper hygiene and periodic dental check-ups. About ten minutes a day will allow you to keep your natural teeth healthy for a lifetime. The oral health care market is a multibillion-dollar-a-year industry. With the increasing proliferation of oral care products available, it is difficult to keep up with all of the possibilities. Knowing some simple facts will make the decision-making process a little easier.

The two major dental conditions which affect most people— dental caries and periodontal disease—are both caused by plaque. Plaque is a collection of various bacteria which take up residence on your teeth and under the gingival tissues. Although it is difficult to see with the naked eye, you can probably find some of this white material by scraping your fingernail along a tooth surface. You can also use plaque-disclosing solution, a pinkish stain that helps reveal the plaque. It is available from your dentist and at most drugstores.

While different bacteria are responsible for caries and the several types of periodontal disease, if the plaque is effectively removed from these areas on a daily basis, the diseases can be controlled and/or prevented. The most common way to control plaque is to remove it mechanically each day. Daily cleaning is necessary because plaque can cause damage only after it becomes organized, a process which takes approximately 12–24 hours.

Another point worth remembering is the effect of advertising. Manufacturers make many claims for their products, and these are occasionally backed up with good scientific evidence. But, for example, claims for plaque reduction are of no use unless there is evidence that the incidence of disease—caries or gingivitis—is reduced as well. For many years, advertisements have touted the ability of one popular pre-brush rinse to reduce plaque, a statement which is true, but have said nothing about a corresponding reduction in inflammation, which the rinse does not affect. By contrast, fluoride-containing toothpastes have been shown to be effective in reducing caries in many well-controlled studies. If you are unsure about a product, ask your dentist.

## Toothbrushing

For people with average manual dexterity, the basic approach to mechanical hygiene is still with a nylon, soft-bristled brush and dental floss. In my opinion, it is better to use a brush with a small head and to concentrate on cleaning one or two teeth at a time instead of trying to do the whole side of the mouth at once. There is no agreement as to the best brush design, hence the proliferation of different brushes available today. Any brush showing the American Dental Association "Accepted" seal on the packaging is acceptable. The ADA Seal of Acceptance signifies that the product, or a similar product, has been tested and proven to be both safe and effective. The correct use of whatever brush you have is more important than its specific design. Incidentally, in cultures where toothbrushes are not available, a wooden chew stick does a very good job in removing plaque.

The brush bristles should be angled toward the edge of the gingiva and the head of the brush moved back and forth in a gentle motion. This will loosen the plaque gently, with the bristles working their way under the margin of the gingiva and between the teeth. The bristles may then be swept toward the occlusal (top) surface of the teeth. This should be done on the facial (outside), lingual (inside), and occlusal surfaces of the

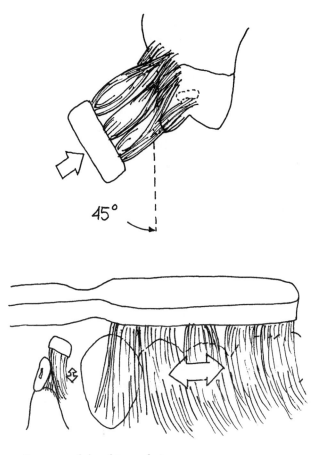

FIG 2–I: Proper tooth-brushing technique

teeth. (Proper brushing technique is illustrated in figure 2–I.)
You should clean slowly, in a systematic manner, starting on one
side of the mouth.

Right-handed people tend to clean the facial (outside)
surfaces of the teeth on their left side first, then bring the brush
toward the front of the mouth. When they turn their hand to
reach the facial surfaces of the teeth on the right, the right

canine is often missed. Use an overlapping stroke in this area to ensure proper cleansing of the canine, first approaching from the left and then starting with the canine when cleaning the right side. Left-handers have the same problem with the left canine. Patients may wonder about the clairvoyance of a dentist who can tell when a patient is left-handed (the left canine being the only tooth with plaque on it).

Brushing can be done first with a wet toothbrush and then again with toothpaste. When brushing the lingual surfaces of your mandibular molars, you will encounter your tongue, which will naturally try to push the toothbrush away from the area you are trying to clean. With a little attention, you can maneuver the brush around this obstruction to clean the lingual surfaces of the teeth. You may also be prone to gag when trying to brush this area. Once again, a small-headed toothbrush will make cleaning easier and more effective.

### Flossing

Brushing is not effective in cleaning the interproximal (side) surfaces of the teeth. For patients without any recession, dental floss is the weapon of choice. The floss is used to wipe the surfaces of the teeth clean of plaque, not just to remove food from between the teeth. About a 3-foot piece of floss should be used for each session. This may seem like a lot until you realize that it costs about 2 cents per piece. Most of the floss should be wrapped loosely around your left middle finger, with a little wrapped around your right middle finger. In this way, as the floss is used, it is taken up on the right finger and unraveled from the left, providing a clean section of floss. Using the middle fingers to hold the floss means that your index fingers and thumbs are free to manipulate the floss as needed. People who wrap the floss around their index fingers then have great difficulty getting the floss where they want it.

The floss is used to clean the interproximal surfaces of the tooth, both above and below the gum line, which the toothbrush

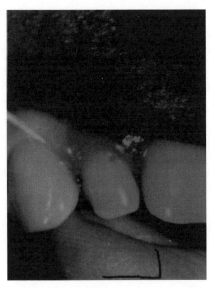

FIG 2–2: Wrapping the floss around the corner of the tooth is necessary for effective plaque removal.

cannot reach. The idea is to wrap the floss around the corners of the tooth and use an up-and-down motion to remove the plaque, as shown in figure 2–2. Many people commonly use the "shoeshine" motion, back and forth, which is not effective. Position the floss between two teeth using your thumbs and index fingers as necessary. Wipe the side of the tooth at least five or six times, as plaque is sticky and cannot be dislodged with one swipe. When one surface is finished, place the floss against the adjacent tooth's surface and repeat the procedure. Two tooth surfaces are cleaned for each placement of floss. Since there is a natural space about 2–3 millimeters deep before the gingiva attaches to the tooth, be sure to carry the floss under the gumline. This will ensure removal of the plaque responsible for causing periodontal disease.

The short answer to the question "What floss should I use?" is any floss that you *will* use. Often, the floss container is a long-forgotten bathroom decoration. Both waxed and unwaxed floss clean effectively when used properly, but unwaxed floss tends to shred more. If you have tightly contacting teeth or rough fillings, waxed floss is preferable. One advantage to unwaxed floss is that it often squeaks when rubbed against a clean tooth surface, whereas waxed floss is noiseless. Floss thickness varies by manufacturer. Here again, the type you use depends on your individual situation, for instance, whether your teeth have tight contacts, fillings, or spacing. Johnson & Johnson floss is relatively thick and difficult to get into tight spots. Floss from Butler and POH is thinner and easier to place in tight areas but is more prone to shredding. There is also flavored floss for those looking for variety in their daily oral hygiene regimen. Some people find floss quite cumbersome to use. A plastic floss holder, which looks like a miniature slingshot, may be helpful. The ease of use is counterbalanced by the device's inability to produce a fresh section of floss for each area, so the floss should be rinsed with water.

If you have any recession of the gingiva between your teeth, the concavities of the tooth roots may be exposed. Floss will not clean these concavities. In this situation, the use of an interproximal brush such as those made by Oral-B and Butler is much more effective, as shown in figure 2–3. These brushes have a handle and interchangeable brush tips. The brush tips have either cylindrical or conical bristle configurations. In either case, the brush is placed between the teeth, with in-and-out and circular motions removing the plaque. The brush should be used from both the facial and lingual directions for maximum effectiveness. A single brush tip will last for varying times depending on the force of your technique. Once the bristles start to compress, change the brush tip. If there are spaces where it is too tight for the interproximal brush to fit, use floss instead.

### Electric toothbrushes

For those who have difficulty handling a manual brush, or who like to have the latest equipment, there are several electric

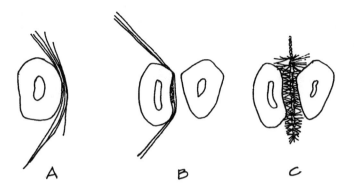

FIG 2–3: A. Floss is effective on teeth with convex root forms. B. Floss cannot remove plaque from root concavities. C. The bristles of an interproximal brush can remove plaque where floss cannot reach.

toothbrushes on the market. It is generally agreed that, all else being equal, powered toothbrushes are more effective than manual ones; however, keep in mind that it is possible to maintain optimal oral health with a manual brush and floss. There is no consensus yet as to which powered brush is best.

The advantages of a powered brush include the availability of different motions in the bristles, and also wider handles, which can be managed by people with arthritis or other dexterity problems. The disadvantages include cost, bulkiness, and the possibility of the motors or charging systems breaking down or wearing out. As with manual toothbrushes, a brush with a small head will allow easier access to hard-to-reach places. It is critical that the bristles be properly angled toward the tooth surfaces, or these brushes will not be of any use at all. In any event, *read the directions* when you purchase a new brush; proper maintenance will significantly extend its life.

### Other oral hygiene aids

If you have a lot of cavities or fillings in your mouth, your dentist may recommend that you use a fluoride gel as part of your oral hygiene regimen. This gel may be applied after brushing and interproximal cleaning. It is usually left on the teeth for one minute and then expectorated. Stannous fluoride is the home fluoride gel most often used both for the control of caries and for tooth sensitivity. Patients with porcelain crowns or composite resin (plastic) fillings should use a neutral sodium fluoride gel, as the stannous fluoride may damage the surface of the restoration.

Toothpastes come in seemingly countless varieties. The basic rule of thumb is to use a fluoride-containing toothpaste with the American Dental Association's Council on Dental Therapeutics Accepted Seal on the label. This seal reads in part "(name of product) has been shown to be an effective decay-preventive dentifrice that can be of significant value when used as directed in a conscientiously applied program of oral hygiene and regular professional care." There are many specialty toothpastes on the market for tooth whitening. Pick one that contains fluoride if you wish to use these products.

Mouth rinses may also be helpful in maintaining your oral health, but only if you pick the right one. Many mouth rinses can freshen the breath; only two major classifications have demonstrated effectiveness in reducing both plaque and gingival inflammation. The first group of mouth rinses contains the detergent chlorhexidine. Chlorhexidine is found in some surgical soaps. In small concentrations, 0.12% in the United States, chlorhexidine has been shown to reduce both plaque and gingivitis over a 6-month period. These are marketed as Peridex® by Procter & Gamble and Periogard® by Colgate. Both are available only by prescription. Chlorhexidine rinses have 3 possible side effects. In many cases, a brownish stain may appear on the teeth, tongue, and tooth-colored composite resin fillings. While the stain is easily removed from enamel, stained roots and composites are much more difficult to clean. You may brush your tongue to help control the brown appearance. The chlorhexidine also has an aftertaste which may be objectionable. This sensation is worsened if you rinse your mouth with water immediately after expectorating the mouth rinse. Some people have also reported a transient change in taste while using the mouth rinse.

The other mouth rinse that has been shown to be clinically effective against gingivitis is that old favorite, Listerine®. The active ingredients in Listerine® include the essential oils—thymol, menthol, and eucalyptol. Among those who use it properly, rinsing for 30 seconds twice a day, there is a clinically significant decrease in gingival inflammation compared to toothbrushing alone or to rinsing with a placebo. While Listerine does not discolor teeth or restorations, it may be uncomfortable to use, especially for the last 10 seconds of a 30-second rinse. Both Listerine and the chlorhexidine products contain significant amounts of alcohol, 26.9% and 18% respectively. Children should only use an alchohol-free mouthwash.

As mentioned in the American Dental Association statement, the rest of your job is to visit your dentist on a regular basis, not just when a raging toothache has you seconds from insanity. Only your dentist can detect minor intraoral changes, which, if left alone, may eventually lead to big trouble but if treated early are easy to manage. The rule of thumb is to have a check-up every 6 months. This can vary depending upon your particular situation. If you are being treated for periodontal disease, your recall interval will be shorter, perhaps 2–3 months between visits. The health of your mouth depends on you. Dentists can repair any damage but their work will only be as good as your ability to prevent any new problems from occurring.

## YOUR DENTIST'S JOB

Dentists have four basic responsibilities regarding your oral health. First, they must complete a thorough examination. Second, they must explain what conditions exist and what the treatment options are, including pros and cons for each. (There may be more than one option available, and often the one chosen will relate to your desires and ability/interest in paying for the proposed treatment.) Third, they must be willing to answer any question that you may have, and fourth, they must be able to provide the proposed treatment in a competent manner or make the appropriate referral. As both the existing conditions and treatment can be complicated, it is imperative that you, the patient, feel comfortable in asking questions. The comment "Do what you think is best, Doc" permits you to abdicate your role as a partner in maintaining your own health.

### Your medical history

The first visit to a dentist usually begins with the completion of a patient demographic and financial information form and a health history questionnaire. The health history questionnaire is very important if you have any medical problems or are taking any medications, either of the prescription or over-the-counter variety. Be sure that you know what medications you are taking and which ones you are allergic to when you arrive for your first appointment. For example, taking a drug as seemingly innocuous as aspirin or one of the many aspirin-related products may cause problems if a tooth must be extracted or a surgical procedure performed. Aspirin, often used by older people to help protect against strokes and heart disease, disrupts the clotting mechanism of platelets and may lead to prolonged bleeding. Even though you may not see the reason for answering a particular question on the questionnaire, each one has a purpose and provides valuable information to the dentist.

There are very few medical conditions which are absolute contraindications for dental treatment, but treatment may need to be altered if you have certain conditions. The presence of a heart murmur or mitral valve prolapse with regurgitation requires the use of antibiotics right before and just after your dental appointment. The heart must be protected from bacteria which enter the bloodstream as a result of dental treatment. Antibiotic coverage for prosthetic joint replacements is somewhat controversial. Orthopedic surgeons usually stand on the side of caution and recommend antibiotic protection. Penicillin and erythromycin are commonly used for prophylaxis against bacterial infections of oral origin. Hypertension (high blood pressure) and diabetes are two other diseases which may require some alteration of treatment. With hypertensive patients, the use of epinephrine-containing anesthetics may be curtailed. Regular monitoring of your blood pressure by the dentist may be in order. Many people who do not know that they have hypertension find out first from routine monitoring by their dentist. Diabetics, especially those on insulin, may need short appointments in the morning. Wound healing in diabetics is often slower, and infections, including intraoral infections, can throw off diabetic control. Epinephrine is also contraindicated for use with certain psychoactive drugs, such as some of those used to treat clinical depression.

**The dental examination**

The dentist should ask you why you have sought treatment. If there is an existing problem, be as comprehensive as possible in relating the location, symptoms, and duration of the problem. The dentist should conduct a complete extraoral and intraoral examination. This includes visual inspection of both the face and neck and palpation of these structures. Beware of any new lumps, bumps, or discolorations in these areas.

Once the extraoral examination is completed, a thorough intraoral examination is performed. Again, this includes visual and manual inspection of the intraoral soft tissues of the cheeks, tongue, floor of the mouth, and oropharynx (back of the throat). A dental explorer—a sharp, pointed instrument placed into the crevices of the teeth—is used to look for the presence of caries. A sticky spot on a tooth may indicate the presence of caries or a deep groove. A transilluminator—a small fiber-optic light wand—may be useful in detecting caries between the teeth. Existing fillings and crowns must also be

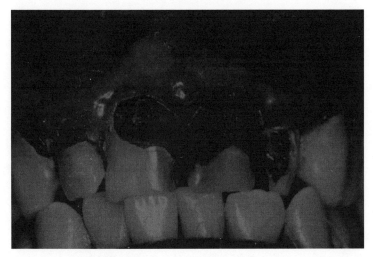

FIG 2–4: Severe dental caries

checked for defects or recurrent decay around the margins of the restorations. Figure 2–4 shows severe caries affecting the maxillary anterior teeth.

In addition to the examination of the oral structures and the teeth, the dentist must perform a thorough periodontal examination. Simply looking at the gingiva and saying everything looks good is not enough. Often, the gingival tissues will not look inflamed or reddened, but there will be severe problems under the gums (see chapter 4). The dentist must use a periodontal probe, a thin instrument with millimeter markings on the shaft, to measure the amount of space from the edge of the gums to where the gingiva attaches to the tooth. Normally, this space will be from 1 to 3 millimeters deep, as shown in figure 2–5. Higher probe readings may indicate any of several possible problems. Bleeding or pus associated with the probing of the gingiva indicates that there is inflammation in the area. A relatively new system, called the periodontal screening and recording (PSR) system, allows the dentist to quickly record these findings. Usually, a PSR score of zero means that there are

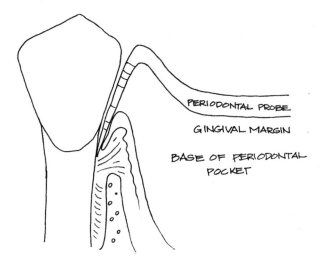

FIG 2–5: The periodontal probe is placed under the gingival margin to measure the depth of the pocket.

no periodontal problems, a score of 1 or 2 means that there may be minor problems, and a 3 or a 4 means that there are more significant problems. The PSR is a simple way for patients to understand their periodontal status as well.

Periodontal problems may show as signs of gingival recession as well as an increase in probing depth. Recession is the shrinkage of the gingival tissues away from the crown of the tooth. This may be caused by periodontal disease, the location of restoration margins or partial denture clasps, or traumatic toothbrushing habits. Tooth size and location in the jawbone may contribute to this recession. At one time, being "long in the tooth" was felt to be a natural part of the aging process. If recession has occurred due to the use of a hard-bristled toothbrush or excessive brushing force, the recession can be stopped by altering the hygiene tools and/or techniques. If recession is due to periodontal disease, the inflammation must be controlled.

The way the teeth come together, or the occlusion, must also be examined. Improper occlusion can lead to the eventual wear or loosening of teeth. New restorations should fit and feel like they belong in your mouth; especially in the case of crowns and dentures, they should not have to "settle in" to fit properly. Restorations that are high will end up putting excessive force on teeth, which may then loosen.

While the clinical examination yields a substantial amount of information, the examination is not complete until an appropriate set of radiographs (X-ray films) is made and interpreted. These films can show damage to the teeth and underlying bone which is not otherwise visible. In some cases, a good panoramic radiograph and bitewing films may be all that is necessary. In other situations, especially when there is periodontal disease present, a full-mouth series of films will show more detail of the condition of the tooth-supporting bone. Figure 2–6 shows the radiographs of two patients, one with minimal bone loss and caries and the other with extensive bone loss and caries.

A few patients object to being exposed to the radiation necessary to obtain these films. While acknowledging their concerns, I ask these patients if they would like me to work on them without wearing my glasses! I also advise these patients that I cannot give them a complete diagnosis of their oral health without the information these films provide, and they have to sign a statement in my chart acknowledging that. All modern radiograph machines have extensive lead shielding to minimize the scatter of X-irradiation. You should also wear a lead apron with a thyroid collar while films are being exposed. Of course, if you are pregnant, the exposure to this and all other forms of radiation should be kept to a minimum. Occasionally, in an emergency situation, one or two films may be made without harm to the fetus.

There are some new advanced technologies which can aid in examination and diagnosis of various dental diseases. They are often used when your dentist cannot arrive at a diagnosis

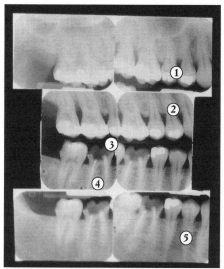

A.

1. Amalgam Restoration

2. Minimal Alveolar Bone Loss

3. Fractured Tooth Crown

4. Gutta Percha Root Canal Filling

5. No Alveolar Bone Loss

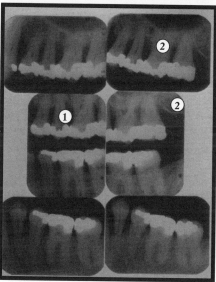

B.

1. Severe Decay Under An Amalgam Restoration

2. Severe Alveolar Bone Loss

FIG 2–6: The radiographs of this patient's mouth show minimal bone loss between the teeth. The lower first molar is fractured, which accounts for the dark appearance of this tooth. B. This patient's radiographs show extensive bone loss and decay.

by more traditional means. In some instances, these diagnostic procedures may be used when treatment is not as effective as anticipated.

Once the examination is complete, the dentist should present you with a complete diagnosis or list of your dental problems. Possible solutions to these problems can then be discussed. As you decide on which course of action to take, it is better not to be penny wise and pound foolish. What seems like more extensive and costlier treatment in the short term may produce more stable and durable results, thus saving time, money, and aggravation, in the long term. (Subsequent chapters will deal with specific dental problems and their solutions.)

## PAYING FOR DENTAL CARE

The financing of dental care is undergoing the same metamorphosis—some would say revolution—that is occurring in medicine. The three major ways of financing dental care are out-of-pocket (dentists call this fee-for-service), some type of dental insurance, and managed care or capitation. In the entire health care financing debate one overarching concept must be kept in mind: you get what you pay for, and in some cases a lot less than what you think you should get regarding your dental plan coverage.

### Fee-for-service

In this system, you, the patient, visit your local dentist. The dentist has specific charges for each service or procedure. The fee has to cover both the direct and indirect expenses incurred during the providing of that service. Direct expenses include the dentist's time and expertise (which many patients forget about), as well as the cost of necessary supplies and materials. Supply costs have skyrocketed over the past few years, as infection control techniques have become significantly more extensive and sophisticated. Indirect expenses include staff salaries, utilities, rent, professional requirements such as license renewal and membership in professional associations, insurance, and other costs of doing business. Dentists set their fees so as to be compensated accordingly. Usually, most general dentists in a certain geographic area have fees at similar levels due to the competition factor. You may not be getting any bargains by going to the least expensive dentist. The costs of doing business will not differ significantly from those of other dentists, so corners will have to be cut somewhere, perhaps in the use of substandard dental laboratories.

Specialists would be expected to have higher fees because of the additional years of training and the increased skill and expertise required of them. Often, specialists are board certified or have diplomate status, meaning that they have demonstrated this expertise to a nationally recognized examining board in their specialty. This requires significant additional time, study, and effort over the completion of specialty training. Not all specialists are board certified. Being "board eligible" or "board qualified" is not the same thing as being board certified. To be sure, non-board-certified specialists can provide the same level of care as boarded specialists, but the boarded individual has demonstrated an additional dedication to excellence.

In any event, in the fee-for-service practice, you are quoted specific fees for specific services and are expected to honor these fees as the services are provided. Many dentists will set up payment plans for extensive, costly treatment.

### Dental insurance

Dental insurance is a form of employee compensation. The dental plan is an agreement between your employer and you. Your dentist has no say in the terms or coverage of your dental plan. Some plans have a fee schedule of their own by which they compensate you for any dental care rendered. This fee schedule may be significantly different from, and is always lower than, your dentist's fee schedule, sometimes to the point that if the dentist charged only those fees to all patients he or she could not afford to stay in business.

You may be responsible for a co-payment, making up the difference from what your plan covers to what the dentist charges. Many dentists contract with insurance plans to accept the plan's reduced fee schedules. But remember, some dentists get squeezed. A single dentist who discounts his fees 20% has to produce 80% more to make up the difference. This is because all of the discount comes out of the dentist's pocket (profit), with the expenses staying the same or increasing! The tendency may then be to cut corners somewhere.

As your dental plan is a contract between your employer and you, your dentist does not have any power to change it. Sometimes the coverage may not be as generous as you would like. Asking dentists to change their reporting so that the plan may pay more is fraud, a criminally punishable offense. Most dentists refuse to do this, while others do acquiesce because they feel the pressure of business. Don't put your dentist in a compromising position.

### Managed care/capitation

These plans make money for the dentist when people sign up for his or her practice but then do not avail themselves of services there. Most managed care/capitation plans are incentives *not* to treat, or to treat in the least expensive way. The fewer services provided, the more money is made by the practitioner or health care group. There is another layer of bureaucracy, one which likes to keep its hands on every last dollar. While many managed care plans look great on paper, mostly because of the supposed decreased cost to you, be very careful to look at the track record of any managed care plan before signing on the dotted line. Some plans cover only very basic services, and practitioners may recommend more expensive services outside the plan to make up for any shortfall from their participation in these plans.

# 3. Dental Caries

Tooth decay, or dental caries, is one of the two most prevalent forms of dental disease, periodontal disease being the other. Four major factors are necessary for caries to occur: a susceptible tooth, presence of acid-producing bacteria, access to fermentable carbohydrates (predominantly sugar) and time. Dental caries is the dissolution of both enamel and dentin by the acid by-products of certain bacteria living on the tooth surfaces. Your mother told you that sugar caused cavities. Actually, the sugar feeds the bacteria which produces the acid which causes cavities. In effect, the minute you finish eating a meal, the meal starts eating your teeth. In addition to that, studies have shown that your mother probably gave you the *Streptococcus mutans*, one of the main bacteria associated with dental caries, in the first place!

Dental caries starts slowly because the process must first work its way through the highly mineralized enamel surface of the tooth. Once the process reaches the less mineralized dentin, the speed of destruction increases. Left alone, the decay may eventually close in on the pulp, causing pain, possible pulpal death, and abscess formation.

## DECAY PREVENTION

Fluoride helps to slow or prevent the decay process by making the enamel less susceptible to acid dissolution. Fluoride is often added to municipal drinking water supplies, and is found in some toothpastes. Even in this era of prevention, approximately 40% of the nation's drinking water is not fluoridated. There is no epidemiological evidence to suggest that fluoride at 1 part per million (ppm) is in any way a health hazard. To be sure, higher concentrations of fluoride, greater than 5 ppm, may cause changes in developing enamel surfaces and extremely high concentrations may be fatal. In addition to the passive use of fluoride in the drinking water, the best way for you to prevent caries is to effectively remove plaque from your mouth on a daily basis (see chapter 2). Interproximal cleaning is as important as smooth surface cleaning. Many cavities start in the contact area between two teeth.

Another factor in caries prevention is the amount and frequency of intake of sugary foods. After eating, the pH, a measure of acidity, decreases around teeth for approximately 20 minutes. A lower pH means greater acid production. This lower pH is eventually raised by the bathing and buffering action of saliva. The sooner you eat, the sooner the pH decreases again. This cycle continues until the decay process starts. One option is to always brush immediately after eating or after drinking sugared beverages. When this is not possible, at least rinse thoroughly with water to decrease the amount of residual sugar in your mouth.

Another method of caries reduction is the use of sealants in the posterior teeth. Sealants are a type of composite resin plastic which is bonded to the chewing surfaces of the molars, as a wood floor would be sealed with polyurethane to protect the wood. The sealant will keep decay from gaining a foothold in the grooves of the molar chewing surface. Sealants are recommended for teeth with deep grooves which are difficult to keep clean. Molars with shallow grooves probably do not need sealants. Teeth which have been in the mouth for several years with no evidence of decay also do not need to be sealed.

There are several habits which are detrimental to healthy teeth. Eating sweetened foods, drinking sugared soft drinks, and chewing sugared gum all contribute to the metabolism of the plaque on your teeth. There is some evidence to suggest that chewing sugarless gum may decrease the incidence of caries. For one thing, the sweeteners in these gums cannot be used by the bacteria to produce acids. Secondly, the stimulation of saliva may have some protective capacity against the formation of a carious lesion by saliva's lavage and buffering actions.

Some foods that are not usually thought of as having high sugar content actually do contain a considerable amount. Raisins and other dried fruits, as well as many non-citrus fruit juices, are high in sugar which can be utilized by the bacteria. Several brands of chewing tobacco contain molasses, basically burnt sugar, to help make the chaw more palatable. Some liquid children's medications are also high in sugar.

Often, babies are put to bed with their bottles. The sugars in milk and fruit juices help to cause rampant caries in the very susceptible maxillary anterior teeth of the child. This "baby bottle caries" or "nursing caries syndrome" can be prevented by placing only water in the baby's crib bottle. The reason the caries progresses so quickly is that the anterior teeth are bathed in the sugar-containing liquid and, because the baby is asleep, the lavage and buffering actions of the saliva are not present. The anterior teeth in these children will decay rapidly, leaving unsightly, sometimes painful tooth stumps. Sometimes these teeth can be fixed with stainless steel crowns, or the teeth may have to be extracted. This syndrome is an unnecessary burden on any child. If the baby is always put to bed with only water in the bottle, or without a bottle at all, that is what he or she will expect.

## WHAT TO DO ABOUT YOUR CAVITIES

### Dental filling materials

Once a tooth is carious, the way it is repaired depends on the location, extent and size of the decay. Three materials are routinely used to fix small-to-moderate-sized cavities: amalgam or alloy, composite resin, and glass ionomer material.

*Dental amalgam.* Dental amalgam or alloy has been in use for approximately 150 years. It is a mixture of silver, copper, tin, mercury and trace amounts of other metals. The advantages of amalgam are that it is easy to use, relatively inexpensive, and very durable. Its major drawback is that its dark silver-gray color contrasts dramatically with the natural appearance of tooth structure. Amalgam is made by mixing shavings of silver, copper, and tin with liquid mercury. The result is a pliable mass which hardens in several minutes. While in the plastic state, the material is placed in the prepared tooth as explained below. The material then hardens, with the maximum hardness achieved after approximately 24 hours.

Almost since it was introduced in the United States in 1833, the use of amalgam has been controversial. Soon after its introduction, some dentists launched a crusade against amalgam, saying that it was no substitute for the use of gold. By 1850, however, amalgam had become a generally accepted dental material, as much for economic as for therapeutic reasons. Today, the controversy rages in a different form. Some people believe that the mercury in amalgam is harmful. While it is true that free, elemental mercury is toxic, there is no evidence that the mercury combined with silver in a hard amalgam restoration, or the trace amounts of mercury liberated from amalgam while a person is chewing, have any deleterious effects. It is impossible to count how many billions of amalgam restorations have been placed over the years and have provided excellent service to patients the world over.

Some dentists preach that the mercury in amalgam is responsible for a whole host of other medical problems. These conclusions may be reached after the patient has been subjected to an expensive battery of tests. The solution, of course, is to have all amalgam restorations removed and replaced. While some restorations may need to be replaced for other reasons, there is no solid evidence that the mercury in set amalgam is responsible for anything.

*Composite resin.* Composite resin is a plastic, tooth-colored material which revolutionized restorative dentistry. Fillings which are virtually undetectable to the naked eye may be placed.

This has vastly improved dentists' ability to create aesthetic restorations for the anterior teeth. Composite resin materials are also used in the posterior teeth, premolars and molars, but are not as durable as amalgam on the chewing surfaces of these teeth. Posterior composites are also very technique-sensitive when used to replace the interproximal surfaces of these teeth. The tooth surface is roughened with acid so that the liquid portion of the composite can flow into these microscopic irregularities. The main composite material, a paste-like substance, is then applied to the tooth. Both the liquid and the paste harden to form a long-lasting filling.

*Glass ionomer.* The third material used often in modern restorative dentistry is glass ionomer, which may be used alone or in conjunction with composite resin. It is tooth-colored but does not have the extensive color-matching capabilities of composite. Glass ionomer has the advantage of chemically bonding to both dentin and enamel. It also has some preventive properties, as it can slowly release fluoride into the surrounding tooth structure.

### How it's done

While you probably have at least one filling in your mouth (most of us do), you may not be familiar with the exact process involved in this type of restoration. After your tooth, and probably your lip, have been made numb with an injection of lidocaine (rather than novocaine, an archaic dental anesthetic), the dentist stretches a latex rubber sheet, known as a dam, over the teeth. Although it may be a bit uncomfortable, the rubber dam allows the dentist to work without worrying about your cheek or tongue being in the way and also helps keep the tooth dry. This dryness is important for the proper placement of amalgam, composite, and glass-ionomer filling materials. In some cases, the dentist may use rolls of cotton to keep the teeth dry while they are beng restored.

Once the rubber dam is placed, the decay is removed with the high-speed handpiece, or drill, the high-pitched instrument which strikes fear in the hearts of dental patients. The decayed tooth structure is removed and the tooth properly shaped to receive the filling material. Sometimes a slower drill, one which has some associated vibration, is used to remove decay close to the pulp. The tooth surface is then conditioned in a specific way to receive the appropriate filling material. If an interproximal surface is being restored, a matrix band—a wall against which the material can be placed—is positioned between the teeth.

The material is then mixed. For amalgams, the metal filings are mixed with the mercury to form the amalgam paste. This paste is then condensed or pressed into the cavity preparation. Enough material is placed to overfill the cavity slightly. While it is still soft, the amalgam is carved with specially designed instruments to re-create the contours of the missing tooth structure. Once this is completed, the matrix band and the rubber dam are removed. The dentist will ask you to bite *gently* on the new filling, checking to see if there are any high spots. These high spots are carved away. The filling should feel like it belongs in your mouth. If it still feels high, do not hesitate to tell the dentist. It is natural, especially after a particularly long appointment or having a large filling done, for a patient to hope that everything is okay, only to go home and feel the high spot. It is better to let the dentist know immediately. High fillings are also prone to fracture, so it is important to get the bite right. Realize that this may be a little tricky if you are still numb.

Composite resin fillings are placed in much the same way, with several modifications. Before the rubber dam is placed, the dentist must pick the proper shade of composite to match your tooth. Once the cavity has been prepared, the surface of the tooth is etched, usually with phosphoric acid. The thin layer of bonding agent, or liquid, covers the tooth surface. The composite resin paste is then placed in the cavity. Unlike amalgam, which starts to set once it is mixed, the composite is light-cured and starts to set only when exposed to bright light. A curing gun is used to harden the resin. The gun may beep every 10 to 20 seconds to alert the dentist to the time of cure.

Large restorations may need to be built up in increments. Once the composite is set, various instruments are used to trim and smooth the final restoration.

The procedures with glass ionomer are similar to those with composite resin. Glass ionomer filling materials are either tooth-colored and often used with composite resin or have silver in them for posterior fillings. Both glass ionomer and composite resin achieve their final set strength right after polymerization.

### Crowns

What happens if the decay is so large that an amalgam or composite resin restoration will not suffice? In these cases, the treatment of choice is an onlay or crown (cap). Onlays and crowns cover the cusps of the tooth and hold the remaining tooth surfaces together. An onlay has margins (edges) located somewhere on the tooth crown so that some of the crown remains visible. A dental crown covers the entire tooth, with the crown margins close to or under the gingival margin. Onlays are usually made from gold alloys, still the finest restorative material known. Gold margins can be made so as to be virtually undetectable to a dental explorer. Of course, gold has the same aesthetic contrast as amalgam, although some people actually prefer to show some gold in their smile.

Both onlays and crowns are made by grinding on the outside of the tooth, not just where the decay is located. Once the tooth is properly shaped, an impression (a mold of the teeth) is made and a stone model poured. The onlay or crown is then constructed in the dental laboratory, where the metal is cast according to the age-old lost wax technique. A crown may have porcelain baked over the metal. The onlay or crown is then delivered to the patient, fitted, adjusted, and cemented. The same rules apply regarding the bite or feel of these restorations. The crown should feel like it belongs to you. Do not let the dentist talk you into allowing the crown to "settle in." Either the occlusion is right or it isn't.

Crowns may be made of three basic materials. Most crowns have a substructure of gold or nonprecious metal with porcelain baked onto the surface of the metal; this is known as the porcelain-fused-to-metal crown or PFM. The metal gives this type of crown strength, while the porcelain matches the shade and contour of the adjacent teeth. For posterior teeth, crowns may be fabricated of all gold or of gold alloy. With these crowns, it is sometimes possible to get a closer marginal fit than with a PFM crown. For anterior teeth where aesthetics may be of major concern, crowns may be made of all porcelain. The new generations of all-porcelain crowns have more strength than their predecessors and superb aesthetic properties.

Just a word about permanence. Amalgams, composites, crowns, and bridges are often called "permanent" restorations. While some may define permanent as eternal, as you should when thinking about your adult teeth, dental permanence approaches the *Webster's New Collegiate Dictionary* definition of "continuing or enduring without fundamental change." The materials with which restorations are made are subject to extremes of heat and cold (such as the drinking of coffee combined with the eating of ice cream) and to chewing forces. Over time, the materials may wear down or fail and the restoration will need to be replaced. The tooth-to-restoration margin is also subject to decay if you allow plaque to accumulate. Although average lifetimes for dental materials have been calculated in the 7–12 year range, some amalgam and gold restorations have been known to last 50 years or more with proper care.

### Root canals

Sometimes the decay has progressed to the point where it gets close to or reaches into the pulp in the center of the tooth. This encroachment may manifest itself as a toothache. If the decay is removed and the pulp has not been physically entered with the dentist's drill, the tooth may be fixed with a conventional restoration. If the decay extends into the pulp, or if there is other evidence that the pulp is damaged or dead, endodontic (root canal) therapy is in order to preserve the tooth.

Root canal therapy involves entering the root canal system which is located in the center of the tooth root. The remaining pulp tissue and/or necrotic debris is removed with special instruments. In some cases, once the canal has been properly cleaned and shaped, the root canal filling material can be placed. This material is usually gutta percha, a type of rubber, which is compacted into the canal system and held in place with a sealer or cement. If the pulp is necrotic or the tooth symptomatic (painful) or infected, it may take two or more visits for the endodontic treatment to be finished.

The general rule of thumb is that there is one canal for each tooth root, but, as rules are made to be broken, often there is an accessory canal in a root. This sometimes presents a challenge because these accessory canals are hard to find and may be narrow, making it difficult to get instruments into the canal for proper cleansing. Once the canals are found, accessory canals are treated in the same way as the main ones.

There is a cult of mythology surrounding endodontic therapy. These procedures are often the targets of jokes, with the mention of a root canal bringing groans from the knowing and nervous laughter from the fearful. The truth is that the majority of endodontic procedures are painless with the appropriate use of local anesthetics. The pain problem arises when the patient has ignored the early warning signs that something may be wrong—intermittent dull pain or throbbing—and waits until the pain is so severe that death seems to be a reasonable alternative. This situation often seems to occur on a Saturday night during the holiday season! In these cases, the pulp is "hot," meaning that it is severely infected and inflamed. In these situations, local anesthetics may mitigate but not completely eliminate the pain. Once the pulp has been removed, the pain and inflammation subside, but getting to that point may be unpleasant.

The other great myth is that root canals "don't work." This claim is often made by people who did not follow through with the recommended treatment that follows the completion of the root canal. Once the pulp has been removed from the tooth, its internal source of moisture is gone. Over time, endodontically treated teeth become brittle. Also, due to the fact that these teeth have large cavities to begin with, there may not be much of the crown remaining. The standard treatment for an endodontically treated tooth is to have the missing parts of the tooth rebuilt with amalgam, composite resin, or glass ionomer. Sometimes some gutta percha is removed and a post is placed in the canal to aid in retention of the buildup. A full coverage crown is then made to restore the tooth to proper form and function.

Failure to follow these recommendations leads to one of two consequences. As the tooth becomes brittle, it is more prone to fracture. If the tooth fractures, sometimes the fracture is favorable, meaning the break is above the gumline, and sometimes it is unfavorable. An unfavorable fracture does not always spell doom for the tooth, but salvation may require some periodontal surgery (crown lengthening) to move the gumline and expose more tooth. In other cases, the tooth must be removed. If a definitive restoration is not placed in the tooth shortly after the root canal is completed, decay may start again, and more tooth is destroyed until it can no longer be fixed by any means.

Teeth which have been endodontically treated are not "dead," only pulpless. The periodontal ligament which holds the tooth to the jawbone is still quite alive. While the pulpless tooth will not have pain of pulpal origin, there is a possibility that pain of PDL origin will occur. This pain is usually associated with abnormal force on the tooth, or occurs if the root of the tooth fractures.

### Repairing decayed primary teeth

Primary teeth can and do occasionally become decayed. As mentioned previously, these teeth provide several important functions for the developing child. In many cases, it is important that a decayed primary tooth is repaired. Leaving the decay untreated may lead to toothache, abscess, or tooth loss. An infected primary tooth may damage the permanent tooth underneath it. The premature loss of a deciduous tooth may cause the other teeth to move, thereby reducing the space available where the permanent teeth erupt. This may eventually result in expensive orthodontic treatment which could have been avoided with some inexpensive treatment earlier.

Primary teeth with small cavities may be restored with amalgam or composite resin. For primary molars with large areas of decay, the treatment of choice may be to remove the pulp tissue by doing a pulpotomy, then placing a medicated filling and a stainless steel crown over the tooth. Anterior teeth may be treated with either stainless steel crowns or with tooth-colored plastic crowns. The restored tooth is then functional and space-holding, and may contribute to aesthetic appeal until it is naturally lost.

If a primary molar has to be removed, be sure to ask your dentist about space maintenance appliances. These appliances, sometimes as simple as a wire loop soldered to an orthodontic band which is then cemented onto a remaining molar, will maintain the appropriate space so that the permanent succedaneous tooth has space to erupt.

## EXTRACTIONS

Certainly maintaining your natural teeth in a state of health and comfortable functioning is your primary goal, as well as dentistry's. Unfortunately, in some cases, because of decay, periodontal disease, or trauma, teeth may have to be removed. Extraction is usually a straightforward affair. After appropriate anesthesia is applied, the tooth is loosened in its socket and then removed with either forceps or elevators. This removal sets up a chain of short-term and long-term events which can affect your oral health for the rest of your life.

### Effects of tooth loss

Let's start with the short-term effects. As the tooth is removed, there will naturally be bleeding from the new wound. If the tissue around the tooth is infected and inflamed, the bleeding may be more pronounced and may occur after you have left the dentist's office. Usually, it can be controlled if you apply pressure by biting on some gauze. If the gauze does not stop the bleeding completely, there are two things you can do before calling your dentist. First, be sure that the gauze has been in the proper position in the first place. Take some clean gauze, dampen it, and bite on it with firm pressure for 30 minutes. This means no talking, eating, drinking, smoking, or spitting. If this does not work, take a tea bag, wet it, and bite on it for 10–15 minutes. The tannic acid in the tea will act as a vasoconstrictor, closing the blood vessels and reducing the bleeding.

If this still does not control things, call your dentist, who no doubt will ask you to do the two things mentioned above. When you say you have already tried these tricks, the dentist will be impressed with your initiative but disappointed as well, for it may mean that he or she will have to see you in the office—now. Do not put this off. If the tea bag trick doesn't work, you could lose a considerable amount of blood in a short time, depending on the extent of the bleeding. Most often, some packing and a suture (stitch) or two are all that is required.

The other major short-term goal is to ensure that the blood clot in the socket remains stable. The clot is the first step in the proper healing of the extraction socket. Sucking, spitting, smoking, and playing with the clot with your tongue can all dislodge it. If the clot is dislodged or disintegrates, a dry socket may result. Although the exact cause of the dry socket is still unclear, the result is not. Pain, sometimes severe, usually occurs and will drive you back to your dentist for relief. The pain comes from exposed nerve endings in the now-uncovered bone. Until your body can wall off this area from underneath the bone lining, the pain will persist. The main treatment for a dry socket is to put in a medicated packing, a procedure which can be quite painful itself. The pain from a dry socket can last from two days to two weeks. Eventually, the uncovered bone will necrose and will be exfoliated from the extraction site in small pieces.

## Post-surgical pain control

Pain accompanies any type of surgical procedure, whether it's periodontal, endodontic, or an extraction. In the past fifteen years there have been great changes in postoperative pain control. Before this time, there were three major classes of analgesics: acetylsalicylic acid (aspirin), acetaminophen, and narcotics. Aspirin and acetaminophen are good for mild pain. Narcotics such as codeine were used for the more moderate-to-severe pain experienced by many surgical patients. The development of the nonsteroidal anti-inflammatory drugs (NSAIDs) has changed postoperative pain management. NSAIDs such as ibuprofen and naproxen have eliminated much of the need for narcotic analgesics. While narcotics act on the central nervous system to deaden the sensation of pain and have accompanying side effects such as nausea and drowsiness, NSAIDs act to stop pain from forming at the local site. Pain is a result of the production of prostaglandins as part of postsurgical inflammation. The NSAIDs block the enzyme cyclooxygenase so that fewer prostaglandins are formed. If you take the appropriate NSAID either before surgery or immediately afterward while you are still numb, the postop pain is significantly diminished. Narcotic medications may still be needed in cases of severe pain, but such instances are much less frequent than they used to be.

## What next?

What happens after the tooth has been removed and initial healing of the socket has occurred? Since the only purpose of the alveolar process of the maxilla and mandible is to house the teeth, once a tooth has been removed, this bone starts to resorb. Resorption is quite variable among individuals but is a universal phenomenon. The resorbed ridge causes aesthetic problems in the maxillary anterior region when fixed bridges are placed and impairs the stability of removable dentures, both partial and complete. The amount of bone remaining on the edentulous ridge is also important in planning the placement of endosseous implants, which are discussed below.

Teeth in general like to be in contact with their neighbors, those to either side as well as those in the opposing arch. When a tooth is lost, the remaining teeth may start to drift into this new space. The drifting causes changes in the tooth-to-tooth relationships and in the bite or occlusion. If the lost tooth is not replaced, these changes can continue until other teeth are in jeopardy of being lost. "Out of sight, out of mind" is not a good axiom to follow once a tooth has been removed.

### Bridges, Partials, and Dentures

There are two ways to replace teeth as long as other teeth remain in the same arch. The most stable replacement is the fixed partial denture, or bridge. A bridge uses crowns as the anchors on the remaining stable teeth on either side of the space, with the replacement tooth or pontic being attached to these anchors. The bridge is cemented to the anchor teeth, as seen in figure 3–1. When properly executed, a bridge feels very similar to natural teeth. The anchor teeth provide the normal tactile sensation to the entire prosthesis. The new bridge provides the maximum stability for the entire occlusion and is able to accommodate occlusal forces approaching those for natural teeth. Bridges are generally made of porcelain-fused-to-metal crowns or are all gold or gold alloy. All-porcelain bridges generally do not have the strength to stand up to heavy occlusal forces.

The other option for tooth replacement when some teeth are remaining is the removable partial denture, what some people call a partial plate or a partial denture. This type of prosthesis uses some of the remaining natural teeth as anchors but is removable. The partial denture will restore chewing function

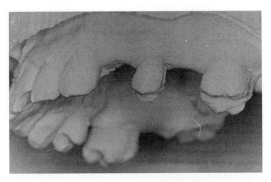

**A.**

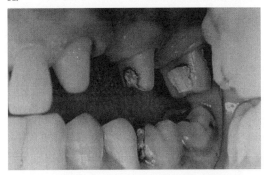

**B.**

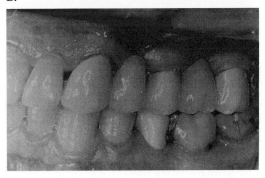

**C.**

FIG 3–1: A. This study model shows the missing teeth on the patient's upper left side. B. The abutment (anchor) teeth have been prepared to receive the crowns. C. The final fixed bridge replaces the first premolar and first molar.

and stability but not to the degree of a fixed bridge. Sometimes the removable partial denture is the only alternative for a person if there are not enough stable teeth to support a bridge.

While a removable partial denture can provide suitable service, it must be evaluated periodically. Over time, the residual jawbone may continue to resorb, changing the underlying support for the partial denture. Subsequently, more force may be placed on the anchor teeth, loosening them. Also, contrary to what you might expect, the anchor teeth for partials are more difficult to keep clean. This makes them more susceptible to caries or periodontal disease.

The final step in the replacement of teeth occurs when a patient is completely edentulous (toothless) in either one or both arches. The removable complete denture is the basic option in this case. The replacement teeth are embedded in a pink acrylic denture which is placed against the residual jaw ridge. The stability of the denture is dependent on the amount of ridge remaining, proper contours of the denture, and the hydrostatic tension created by placing one wet surface against another (try separating two wet pieces of glass without sliding them against each other).

A maxillary complete denture is relatively stable. The extension of the denture over the entire expanse of the palate helps keep the denture stable and retentive even when there is little residual ridge on which the denture can rest. The mandibular arch can be much more problematic. The mandibular denture is inherently less stable because of the horseshoe shape of the mandible and the decrease in surface area on which the denture rests. A patient with a severely resorbed mandibular ridge may not be able to wear a lower denture successfully. The denture can be dislodged by chewing forces which would not disturb a maxillary complete denture. Several studies suggest that even the best-made complete dentures can only generate approximately 20% of the chewing force of natural teeth. The bottom line is, if given the choice, you should do anything you can to save at least some of your mandibular teeth!

# DENTAL IMPLANTS

Dental implants have become quite popular over the past ten years, although the general idea of implants is not new. The first specimen of a successful endosseous (within bone) implant is believed to be one which was discovered in Honduras in 1931. This piece of mandible had three tooth-shaped pieces of shell in line with the remaining teeth. Radiographs showed that the jawbone grew around the shell "implants" in much the same way that bone grows around modern titanium implants. Dating from 600 A.D., the specimen was probably Mayan.

Modern implantology is based on work that started about 30 years ago in Sweden, in which some novel concepts of implant design and placement were employed. In essence, a titanium screw or slug is screwed or tapped into an osteotomy site (hole) in the bone. The implant is covered with the gingiva and left undisturbed for several months to allow the jawbone to grow around the surface of the implant and hold it in place. Once proper bone healing has occurred, the implant is uncovered and the proper attachments are screwed into the top of the implant, as illustrated in figure 3–2. These attachments replace the missing teeth or provide the anchors upon which a complete denture sits. Implants may be used to replace a single tooth or to support a removable complete denture, short bridge, or an entire arch of teeth.

It would be nice if implantology were as easy to carry out as it is to write about. Many factors contribute to successful implant therapy. First and foremost, it must be remembered that the implant patient is a dental failure, whose natural teeth have been lost for some reason. This reason must be discovered and the cause(s) eliminated or controlled. In cases where trauma has caused the loss of teeth, this is an easy matter. When teeth have been lost due to neglect, the patient must understand in no uncertain terms that implants can and will fail if not cared for properly. The same bacteria which cause periodontal disease can cause inflammation around implants, resulting in their loosening

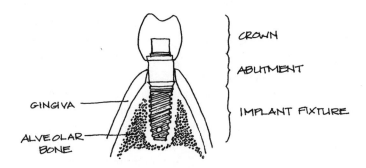

CROWN

ABUTMENT

IMPLANT FIXTURE

GINGIVA

ALVEOLAR BONE

FIG 3–2: The anatomy of an implant restoration.

and necessitating removal. Implants need the same daily ritual of proper oral hygiene as their natural counterparts. Those considering it should ask themselves: if I didn't take care of my teeth, will I take care of my implants?

Biologically, your bone is the key to implant success. All bone is not created equal. The bone in the anterior region of your mandible is thick and dense, ideal bone for implant placement. The bone in the posterior of your maxilla is thin and sparse, much less suitable for implant placement. The amount of bone is also critical. Implants generally must be at least 10 millimeters long and 3.0 millimeters wide to be successful. There must be a sufficient volume of bone to accommodate these dimensions without the implant violating vital structures such as nerves, blood vessels, or the maxillary sinus. Your dentist, or the surgeon who will be placing the implants, may request that a CT scan be made of your jaws. This supplies an accurate picture of both the amount and quality of your bone, as well as the relative locations of those vital structures to be avoided. In some instances, additional bone can be grown or structures such as nerves or the floor of the maxillary sinus can be moved out of the way. Be sure that any complicated implant procedures (are there any other kind?) are done by experienced operators.

There must be excellent communication and coordination between the periodontist or oral surgeon who is placing the implants and the dentist who will be restoring them. Inadequate communication may lead to poorly placed implants which cannot then be restored due to their location or angulation. There is no question that many people have had their lives significantly improved by dental implant therapy. Those who cannot wear a conventional mandibular complete denture can have a stable, confidence-restoring prosthesis supported by the implants. When replacing a single tooth, the use of an implant may obviate the necessity of grinding on two healthy adjacent teeth to support a conventional fixed bridge. An implant-supported fixed bridge may be fabricated where only a removable partial denture could be used before.

As noted previously, there is no such thing as eternal permanence in dentistry. Implants, and especially the attachments to the implants which constitute the replacement teeth, can break. In controlled studies, some current designs of endosseous implants have been functioning in patients' mouths for over 30 years. Not all implant restorations have lasted that long, some not even 30 months. There is still much to be learned about implantology, as dentists stretch the envelope to treat difficult situations in ways they could not have dreamed of only a few years ago.

## LOOKING YOUR BEST

As mentioned in the introduction, one of the major functions of the mouth is to provide you with a smile. While the smile is universal, aesthetic concepts associated with it have changed over the ages. Leonardo da Vinci's *Mona Lisa* and Madonna both have attractive smiles, but their faces are quite different, and the cultural context in which they appear has changed.

One constant goal of people who want to improve their smile is to have "white" teeth. In fact, teeth are not white in the starched-shirt sense but exhibit shades of white, yellow, and other characteristics blended together. This is apparent in the case of some celebrities whose teeth are too white and too bright to be natural.

A variety of techniques may be used to change the appearance of teeth. Bleaching, either in a dentist's office or at home, is the simplest way to change the surface color of the teeth. Most bleaching techniques use a peroxide-containing compound as the base, combined with catalysts or other substances to lighten the teeth. The peroxide is activated with either heat or light from a bright lamp or perhaps a laser. The at-home bleaching technique is simpler. A mouth guard (similar to an athlete's) is filled with the bleaching peroxide and worn while you sleep. Bleaching works best on extrinsic stains or discoloration close to the surface of the tooth. Deep discoloration, such as that caused by the ingestion of the antibiotic tetracycline while the teeth are forming, is best covered over by other methods. Care must be taken not to get the bleaching agents on the gingival tissues, which could result in inflammation and ulceration. Over time, if there is fading or restaining, the bleaching will have to be repeated.

Tooth discoloration may be masked and teeth may be reshaped through the use of plastic composite resin veneers, porcelain veneers, or full porcelain crowns. The composite veneers have been in use for many years. While more economical than the other options, composite veneers cannot achieve the same natural appearance as porcelain and are subject to wear and stain accumulation over time. Porcelain veneers require a minor amount of reshaping of the visible surface of the tooth to create space for the veneer. An impression (mold) is made of the teeth and the veneers are custom made by a dental laboratory technician. The veneers are then attached to the prepared tooth surfaces with tooth-colored cements.

Porcelain crowns have been used for many years to change the appearance of the teeth, especially front teeth. These crowns may be made in several ways, ranging from the strongest to the most aesthetic. The strongest crowns have a metal or gold base which reinforces the porcelain. While these crowns have the greatest strength, there is a possibility that the metal margin may be visible through thin gingival tissue. Gingival recession will make the metal margins visible, which may be unsightly. All-porcelain crowns provide the best appearance but are not as strong as porcelain and metal crowns, which are perfect in the anterior part of the mouth where the patient does not place severe forces on the teeth. A suitable compromise for the gaining of both strength and aesthetics is the "collarless" crown. These crowns have a metal structure except on the visible margins. The crown-tooth interface looks more natural than it does with the porcelain-metal crown.

While a significant amount of time, effort, and money may be invested in aesthetic anterior crowns or veneers, the overall natural appearance is only as good as the health of the gingival tissues. Maintenance of proper, atraumatic oral hygiene is imperative to preserve the overall aesthetic effect. Healthy, pink tissues add to the natural appearance of well-done anterior aesthetic procedures.

# 4. Periodontal Disease

Periodontal disease comprises two main categories: gingivitis and periodontitis. Gingivitis is inflammation of the gingival (soft) tissue only. It is indicated by swelling of the gingiva, erythema (redness), and bleeding when the gingiva is brushed or probed. Most people, probably more than 95%, have had gingivitis at some time during their lives.

Periodontitis is often the silent destroyer. The gingival inflammation spreads so that the bone which supports the teeth starts to deteriorate, as seen in figure 2–6. In the early stages, this deterioration is unknown to the patient. There is no pain, and the surface signs are similar to those of gingivitis. Over time, there is deepening of the pockets around the teeth, perhaps some recession of the gingiva, and eventual loosening of the teeth when enough bone is lost.

It is common for patients to state that they did not know anything was wrong; they may have been getting regular dental checkups, during which the condition was undetected. This underscores the importance of using the periodontal probe to examine the depths of the pockets during the initial or recall examination. The use of good radiographs also provides information about the amount of bone loss.

Both gingivitis and periodontitis are caused by that old enemy, bacterial plaque. Different bacteria in the plaque are responsible for gingivitis and the various forms of periodontitis. In most instances, identifying the specific plaque microorganisms is not necessary for successful treatment of periodontal disease. What is necessary is the removal of the harmful plaque on a daily basis, as discussed in chapter 2. Other factors can contribute to the progression of periodontal disease. Smoking has been shown to have an adverse affect on periodontal health. In women, changes in hormone levels can increase gingival inflammation. Some women experience pregnancy gingivitis—severe inflammation of the gums—due to the overgrowth of certain bacteria which feed on hormones secreted in the fluid from the gingiva.

## WHAT HAPPENS?

Periodontal disease is basically an inflammatory reaction to the plaque which collects on your teeth and under your gums. In health, specific bacteria, usually those which are positive for the Gram's stain (a special stain which is used to help identify bacteria) are aerobic (can use oxygen) and stationary. As plaque collects over a period of days or weeks, the characteristics of the specific bacteria change. The bacteria within the plaque become Gram negative, are strictly anaerobic (cannot survive in the presence of oxygen), and are more motile. These newer bacteria include rods and spirochetes, some of which can invade the connective tissue of the gingiva. These bacteria are much more virulent, and, when placed anywhere else in the body besides the mouth, can cause life-threatening infections. In effect, periodontal disease is the body's reaction to these highly virulent bacteria. The periodontium is destroyed in the body's attempt to protect the rest of itself from these organisms.

As the plaque collects on your teeth, the mass absorbs the minerals from your saliva. Over time, the soft plaque mass uses these minerals to harden into dental calculus, or tartar. While calculus is not harmful in itself, it provides a lovely ecological niche in which plaque thrives. When allowed to grow unimpeded, it will eventually become an unsightly irritant to the gingival tissues. The treatment of periodontal disease includes the removal of calculus, as well as of plaque.

The Gram negative organisms in plaque trigger inflammation in the gingiva and periodontium. Neutrophils (polymorphonuclear leukocytes or PMNs), the first line of defense of the immune system, are attracted to the area of plaque accumulation. These cells are equipped to engulf and destroy many of the accumulated bacteria. In the process, the PMNs release a cascade of enzymes which destroy the connective tissue of the gingiva. The PMNs are joined by macrophages, the other cell type found in early stages of inflammation. The macrophages produce a variety of substances, cytokines, which both stimulate PMNs to perform various functions and trigger other parts of the immune response. Eventually, plasma cells, which make antibodies specific for each bacteria present, arrive on the scene. In what is literally a battle of good vs. evil, the connective tissue and the bone which supports the teeth are the main casualties.

In ways that are not clearly understood, this process undergoes periods of intense activity followed by peaceful intervals. The loss of connective tissue and the progressive deepening of the periodontal pockets continue for a time and then cease. Various events may start the process anew. A general decrease in the immune resistance of the host, such as the contracting of flu or other illness, may tip the scales to start the destruction again. Food wedged between the teeth, a popcorn hull caught under the gingiva, or a new filling with a rough margin can all act as stimulants. There is still no clear predictor for further destruction except for the bleeding of the gums that goes along with the inflammation.

As the inflammatory process continues, the destruction spreads from the connective tissue of the gingiva to the alveolar bone which supports the teeth. As this bone is destroyed, the teeth may become loose and start to change position. When this occurs, the periodontitis has progressed to an advanced stage. All is not lost, but delay in seeking attention will result in tooth loss. One thing to keep in mind, even when teeth can be saved from advanced periodontitis, is that the decisions regarding restoration often hinge on how stable the remaining teeth will be.

You may be able to detect some of the signs of periodontal disease yourself, the most common being the "pink toothbrush syndrome." This, obviously, indicates gums which bleed when you brush your teeth. Often, this is the *only* sign you have that something is wrong. Many people incorrectly assume that a little bleeding is natural, usually because their gums have always bled when they cleaned their teeth. Bleeding is a sign of inflammation, but it does not signify the extent of the periodontal problem. You may also notice that your gums are red. Here, too, this redness is not a measure of the severity of the problem. When you notice that your teeth are starting to drift around, you can be sure that the problems are getting to the severe stage.

Bad breath has also been associated with periodontal disease. The sulfur compounds which are produced by biologic debris collecting in your mouth cause halitosis. Mouth rinses may camouflage the odor temporarily, but only a thoroughly clean mouth will not offend.

## TREATMENTS

What should you do when you think you have periodontal disease, or pyorrhea, as it is sometimes called? A visit to your general dentist or periodontist for a thorough examination is in order. As mentioned in chapter 2, this examination will include measuring your periodontal pockets with a probe marked in millimeter increments. Healthy tissue will have readings in the 1–3 millimeter range with no bleeding. Gingivitis is marked by bleeding on gentle probing, with possibly some slight increase in probing depth. Periodontitis is marked by probing depths from 4 millimeters and higher, with bleeding on probing. There may also be some recession of the gingival margin away from the cementoenamel junction, exposing more of the tooth. In either situation, you are dealing with decreased support for the teeth in question. There may also be some increased pocketing in the furcation area between the roots of the molars. The teeth have increased mobility, and may have moved from their original position.

Of course, each individual situation will require a customized plan; what follows is a general outline regarding treatment of periodontal disease. You, the patient, are an active participant in this treatment. What your general dentist, periodontist, or dental hygienist does with you, for you, and to you is only as successful as what you do for yourself on a daily basis.

First and foremost, the plaque which causes the disease must be thoroughly removed on a daily basis for inflammation to be properly controlled. Your therapist can give you specific guidelines on the use of a brush, floss, interproximal brush, and other hygiene aids. Plaque does not know that you are tired or under stress from work or family life, and does not go on vacation when you do. Be sure to spend the 10 minutes each day necessary to do a good job, preferably before you retire for the evening, although morning is acceptable if that is more convenient.

Scaling and root planing—the scraping of your teeth and under the gums—constitute the basic therapeutic approach to controlling inflammation by removing plaque and calculus. Your dentist and hygienist will accomplish this either with hand instruments, an ultrasonic cleaner, or both. An ultrasonic cleaner, commonly called a Cavitron®, which is actually a specific brand of ultrasonic device, uses high frequency vibrations to blast the calculus from your teeth. The copious amounts of water which accompany this procedure are needed to cool the ultrasonic handpiece.

This scaling and root planing may be accomplished over several visits. It may be necessary to anesthetize the quadrant in which the scaling will be done because of the possible discomfort associated with the procedure. In difficult cases, scaling is a time-consuming process. Repeated visits allow the therapist to ascertain the progress of healing and the discovery of calculus missed at the first visit. Scaling is done most effectively in pockets of 5 millimeters or less, with the effectiveness decreasing considerably in pockets of 7 millimeters or greater. In these instances, other means may be employed to achieve clinical success.

Scaling and root planing have several results, some of which are desirable and some of which are not. The removal of plaque and calculus brings with it a reduction in inflammation, bleeding, and perhaps a decrease in pocket depth as well. Depending on the amount of edema (swelling), the gingiva may shrink and recede as the inflammation subsides. This will expose more tooth structure, which may be aesthetically objectionable in the anterior part of the mouth. Unfortunately, this may be biologically unavoidable and is the price paid for having the disease in the first place. Recession may also make the teeth sensitive to cold and sweets. This sensitivity is usually transient in nature and often controlled with the use of a desensitizing toothpaste.

Once the scaling is completed, the teeth are selectively polished to remove any stain and loose plaque. This is done with a rotating rubber cup and a mild abrasive paste. Most people equate polishing with a cleaning. Polishing may be effective in treating mild gingivitis but is not effective in treating periodontitis. Most patients, even after having undergone several appointments of scaling, want to know when they will be getting their teeth cleaned. From the therapist's viewpoint, the scaling is the cleaning.

## ABOUT ANTIBIOTICS

Since periodontal disease is primarily an infection most likely caused by Gram negative bacteria, it is reasonable to wonder why these infections cannot be treated with antibiotics as other bacterial infections are. The nature of the disease sheds light on the answer. It is well established that most cases of adult periodontitis, the most common form, respond well to the mechanical therapy of scaling, root planing, and routine plaque removal. Most of the bacteria which cause this infection live in the pocket itself and can therefore be removed by scaling, root planing, brushing, and flossing. Many studies have shown that, over time, the clinical result would be the same whether or not antibiotics were used. This being the case, antibiotics are not the treatment of choice in adult periodontitis. The possibility of antibiotic resistant strains of bacteria emerging as a result of prolonged antibiotic therapy is always a threat. As will be seen later, antibiotics may be used if adult periodontitis becomes refractory, meaning that it does not respond to conventional therapy.

There is a unique form of periodontitis, juvenile periodontitis, which is marked by an infection with *Actinobacillus actinomycetemcomitans*, a virulent Gram negative rod. These bacteria invade the gingival connective tissues as well as populating the pocket. No amount of scaling and root planing will eradicate these bacteria, nor will surgery alone. Tetracycline or one of its derivatives is used to eliminate the *Actinobacillus actinomycetemcomitans* from the gingival tissues in juvenile periodontitis patients.

As the name suggests, juvenile periodontitis affects children and adolescents. There is rapid destruction of the bone surrounding the permanent incisors and permanent first molars, the first permanent teeth to erupt in the mouth. This severe destruction may be attributable to a hyperimmune response by the patient's macrophages. These cells secrete unusual amounts of cytokines which affect neutrophils and other players in the immune response in various ways. The result is a "suped-up" response to the infection with accompanying tissue destruction. Over time, the body produces antibodies against *Actinobacillus actinomycetemcomitans* which protect the later erupting teeth from colonization by the bacteria.

Juvenile periodontitis is the one form of periodontitis with a clear genetic link. Family studies have shown that susceptibility to the disease, and the associated changes in the immune response, are inherited. While its passage from one generation to the next has been established, the exact location of the gene or genes on which chromosome has yet to be confirmed.

One other form of periodontitis in which systemic antibiotic treatment is indicated is refractory periodontitis. This type of periodontitis is often diagnosed through a process of elimination, meaning that it has not responded to conventional forms of therapy, including surgery. In these situations, plaque samples are taken from the deepest pockets, or from pockets which continue to have bleeding and pus formation. Using either microbial culturing or DNA probe technology, the bacteria in the pocket can be identified. Appropriate antibiotic therapy can then be instituted.

A variety of antibiotics, and combinations thereof, may be used to treat refractory periodontitis. Some commonly used antibiotics include Augmentin® (a combination of amoxicillin and clavulanic acid), ciprofloxacin, clindamycin, metronidazole, and tetracycline. Specific regimens depend on the bacteria present.

While culturing can identify which bacteria are present in a pocket, there is no definitive proof that these bacteria caused the disease. It is a supposition that the presence of putative pathogens indicates that antibiotics be used. In addition, the bacteria in the sample must be viable when the sample arrives at the microbiology laboratory for culturing to be of any use. DNA probe analysis is more restrictive in identifying the bacteria present. While this technique does not need live bacteria, probes only to the usual suspects have been developed. A periodontal infection by an organism for which a probe is unavailable would not be detected.

A word of caution to women who use oral contraceptives and must take antibiotics for periodontal (or other) reasons. Certain forms of birth control medications are metabolized to their active state by bacteria in the small intestine. Antibiotic usage may disrupt the normal bacterial flora of this area, which could alter the effectiveness of the contraceptive. Although this relationship between antibiotics and oral contraceptive effectiveness is controversial, it is advisable that alternative forms of birth control be used, not just during the course of antibiotics but for the remainder of that cycle.

Another caveat for women who use antibiotics is the possibility of vaginitis. Those who have problems with *Candida* infections should be forewarned that these infections can flare up with antibiotic usage. The antibiotics wipe out normal bacteria in the vagina, thus allowing the *Candida* to overgrow.

There may be a time when conventional therapy works quite well except in one or two isolated pockets. These areas may not be amenable to surgical therapy, and systemic antibiotics may not be indicated either. In these instances, it would be nice to have a locally delivered antibiotic which could eradicate the infection.

As of this writing, several companies are working on both delivery systems and antibiotic combinations that can be placed in isolated pockets. To date, only Procter and Gamble, in association with Alza Laboratories, has been able to market a tetracycline which can be delivered locally to the site. Actisite® is a tetracycline-impregnated, nonresorbable vinyl ethyl acetate fiber which can be placed in an infected pocket. Over a 10-day period, the tetracycline is slowly released from the fiber to eliminate the bacteria. The fiber is then removed and the pocket allowed to heal. Healing continues over a 2-month period with final pocket reduction seen at the end of that time.

Actisite® has been marketed for use in isolated 5–8 millimeter pockets and for use in sites which have developed problems during maintenance. Clinical experience has shown that it does not always work (neither does anything else), but significant improvements can be obtained. Several companies are on the brink of marketing similar devices which resorb in the periodontal pocket and do not have to be removed.


## PERIODONTAL SURGERY

What scares many patients about periodontal therapy is the prospect of having to undergo surgery. If you do a good job of controlling plaque and do not have any deep pockets, you should have nothing to worry about. For those who may find themselves facing such a prospect, perhaps some background information will be helpful.

Scaling and root planing form the backbone of conventional therapy. As pockets deepen past about 5–6 millimeters, the effectiveness of scaling diminishes. In 10-millimeter pockets with furcation involvement, complete removal of calculus is virtually impossible scaling into a closed periodontal pocket. Without this removal of calculus and plaque, the pocket will not heal. The primary reason to perform periodontal surgery is to move the gingiva out of the way so that the calculus can be more readily removed. Everything else is secondary to this goal.

There are many kinds of surgical flap procedures, but most fall into one of three general types. As noted, surgery is done to expose the teeth so that the calculus can be removed. The gingiva is then replaced in approximately the same position from which it was taken. In the presence of deep pockets and irregularly shaped bone, the bone may be reshaped and the gingiva placed against it. This may result in the teeth appearing longer after healing, but any deep pockets will have been eliminated.

The third type involves growing back some of the bone, cementum, and periodontal ligament which has been destroyed by the disease. This regeneration is the future of periodontal therapy. Currently, regeneration is achieved through the use of a surgical flap to gain access to the teeth and bone. Then, bone grafting materials such as demineralized freeze-dried bone allograft or some artificial bone substitutes are used to stimulate or encourage new bone growth. A membrane barrier, such as one made from Teflon® or some resorbable polymers, is used to block unwanted cells from growing in the regeneration site. Over time, bone and other desirable tissues will form and regenerate support for the teeth.

Periodontal regeneration has been an active area of research for the past 30 years. The current thrust is to develop ways in which natural growth factors can be introduced into a site of periodontal destruction and new bone can be grown in a predictable fashion. Current techniques for regeneration are only predictable in sites with certain patterns of bone destruction. Not all bone destroyed by disease can be rebuilt.

Another area of development is in the rebuilding of a residual jaw ridge where the teeth have been lost. In the maxillary anterior region, ridge resorption and destruction make the fabrication of a bridge that looks natural very difficult, if not impossible. By using the patient's own connective tissue, this deficient ridge can be rebuilt so that the replacement teeth, the pontics, look like actual teeth growing out of the gumline. In this case, the bridge looks like real teeth instead of what it is. For those who are conscious of aesthetics in such situations, these techniques make all the difference.

The final word on periodontal therapy is that prevention is the key. The best defense is never to get periodontal disease in the first place. Once you have it, even though the disease can be controlled with good therapy, excellent oral hygiene, and a regular maintenance schedule with your dentist, you will always be susceptible to a recurrence of disease. Establishing and maintaining a regular schedule of visits to your dentist is critical. Studies suggest that no matter what type of therapy is performed, it is only as successful as the maintenance program. Don't get lazy once the disease is under control; periodontal health is a lifelong commitment.

# 5. Crooked Teeth and Orthodontics

Chances are good that either you or your children (or both) have had a long-standing and expensive relationship with an orthodontist. While your 13-year-old daughter may just want straight teeth for the prom, there are some very good health reasons for having straight teeth as well. A pleasing smile certainly affects a person's sense of self. Straight teeth are easier to keep clean and less prone to collect debris and plaque than crooked teeth. Teeth that are in proper alignment function better and provide more sound support for the occlusion. Given the benefits, orthodontic treatment is a better investment than a luxury car or a big-screen television.

Several factors conspire to create a mouthful of crooked teeth. As humans have evolved, overall jaw size and arch length have decreased. Often, children inherit their father's teeth and their mother's jawbone structure. This can mean that the teeth are too big for the alveolar housing—hence, the crowding. In certain races and ethnic groups, malocclusion due to crowding is more the rule than the exception. The opposite can also happen, so that spaces will occur between teeth because the mother's teeth are in the father's jaws. In rare cases, teeth are congenitally missing; unfortunately, this does not seem to occur in those who are susceptible to crowding in the first place.

Good orthodontic therapy may have to start early, sometimes as soon as the satisfactory eruption of the permanent first molars has taken place. If your general dentist notices that your child has unusually small jaws, you should be aware that there are techniques to help redirect the growth of these bones. For instance, sometimes the roof of the mouth is constricted, leaving the maxillary arch too narrow. A dentist using a palatal expansion appliance can stretch the maxilla by widening the midpalatal suture. This type of treatment, called interceptive orthodontics, must be done before the suture starts to calcify. The purpose of preventive orthodontics, as the name suggests, is to try to prevent occlusal problems from occurring in the first place. The use of space maintainers when primary teeth are lost prematurely may prevent crowding and allow the permanent tooth to erupt properly.

Severe crowding can also be avoided by what is termed serial extractions. When a tooth size/arch size discrepancy has been detected, the first permanent premolars may be removed as they erupt into the mouth, thus creating space where the rest of the teeth can line up in a more orderly fashion. Subsequent orthodontic treatment may be less complicated or of shorter duration.

Orthodontic tooth movement is accomplished by the placing of a controlled force, through the use of brackets, wires, springs, and elastics, on the teeth. Occasionally, a headgear is used to direct both tooth movement and skeletal growth. As light, directed forces are applied to teeth, the alveolar bone on the pressure or compression side will begin to resorb. Bone on the tension side, away from the directional force, will be formed maintaining the overall shape of the tooth socket. The patient will experience pain when the force is initially applied. Within 2 to 3 days after an adjustment visit, the body begins to accommodate to this force and the pain diminishes.

Movement of teeth through bone is a slow process. Good compliance with the orthodontist's directions are critical to timely treatment. Failure to change elastics as directed, to keep the teeth and gums as clean as possible, or to return to the office for repair of a broken appliance may significantly delay completion of treatment. At the end of treatment, any prescribed retainers must be faithfully worn, or teeth will tend to move back to their original locations. Poor oral hygiene while one is wearing braces may lead to severe decay around the appliances.

Orthodontic therapy is not for children only. Over the past decade, significantly greater numbers of adults have sought orthodontic care. While the biomechanics are similar in adults and children, there are several major differences. In adults, there can be no redirection of skeletal growth, as this aspect of life is finished. Adults may also have some overlying TMD problems (or "TMJ," as it is popularly known; see chapter 6) which should be addressed to the greatest extent possible before treatment. The specter of periodontitis is real in adult orthodontic patients. While it seems that adolescents can practice poor oral hygiene and end up only with gingivitis, severe periodontal destruction awaits the adult patient with poor plaque control or underlying undiagnosed periodontitis. Final posttreatment retention may be more complicated. In some cases, permanent retention is indicated.

# 6. What Else Can Go Wrong?

Chapters 3 and 4 dealt with dental disease of a chronic nature. However, both caries and periodontal disease can progress to the point where a dental emergency, usually in the form of a toothache or abscess, occurs. Other problems which can occur in your mouth include difficulties with wisdom teeth, ulcerations, malignant tumors, and halitosis (bad breath).

## DENTAL EMERGENCIES

### Toothaches and abscesses

As mentioned previously, most dental problems are painless, at least initially. Dental caries will progressively destroy the tooth structure without giving you any clue as to what is going on. Eventually, the decayed tooth may become sensitive to cold, hot, or sweets due to initial irritation of the tooth pulp. Even then, the discomfort may not be enough to cause a person to seek attention. The tooth may be sensitive for a while and then become comfortable once again. The pain may return, somewhat more pronounced than before but still not severe. Sooner or later, the decay and the bacteria which cause the decay will reach the pulp of the tooth. As the nerve in the pulp becomes irreversibly inflamed or begins to die, the toothache becomes more constant and involves greater amounts of pain. If the pulp dies and becomes infected, an abscess, with associated pain and swelling, may result. The tooth may feel high to the bite and may loosen in the socket.

Treatment for a tooth such as the one described in the preceding scenario depends on what stage has been reached by the time the dentist is seen. If it is not possible to get immediate treatment, analgesics such as the nonsteroidal anti-inflammatory drugs and/or antibiotics may be the treatment of choice. In its early stages, even with some mild sensitivity, the decay can be removed and a restoration placed in the tooth. Once the tooth becomes painful during chewing, awakens you from a sound sleep, or hurts for no apparent reason, endodontic therapy will be necessary. Even if the tooth is abscessed and there is swelling present, many times it can be saved. Sometimes the swelling will be treated with antibiotics or the swollen area incised to allow the collected pus to drain away. Sometimes the body forms a small channel in the gums, a fistula, to allow the pus to drain from the abscess. Once this drainage starts, the pain usually diminishes greatly. If the decay has progressed to the point where the tooth cannot be restored, or if there has been significant destruction of the surrounding alveolar bone, the tooth may have to be extracted.

While many abscesses are caused by a decayed tooth, there are also periodontal abscesses which are associated solely with the gingiva and the underlying bone. Most periodontal abscesses are caused by the entrapment of food particles, such as popcorn husks, or by calculus beneath the gingiva. An abscess forms when the pus associated with the infection cannot drain through the pocket. In these cases, the tooth may be sore or loose, but the infection is confined to the soft tissue and adjacent bone. Most periodontal abscesses can be treated by draining the pus and cleaning the pocket of the offending material. Antibiotics are occasionally used to treat an abscess of strictly periodontal origin.

Things get more complicated when there are both endodontic and periodontal problems with which to contend. The diagnostic challenge for the dentist is determining to what degree the pulp or inflamed periodontium contributes to the abscess. In a true combined lesion, the endodontic therapy is finished first, allowing the body several weeks to heal. Any remaining periodontal problems are then addressed. In some cases, the endodontic problem actually causes the periodontal problem as well. As the root canal therapy is completed, the gingival problem disappears.

## Traumatized and avulsed teeth

Teeth may be traumatized or avulsed (knocked out), during various kinds of mishaps, including auto accidents, sports injuries, violent attacks, and general horsing around. If a tooth is hit but not dislodged, the crown will turn gray over time. This is due to the breakdown of hemoglobin within the tooth; the trauma will have caused some minor bleeding in the pulp, and the blood will seep into the tubes in the dentin. Such a condition is especially disconcerting to the parents of a toddler who develops a darkened tooth following a fall.

When a tooth is completely lost, it may have been knocked cleanly from its bony housing, or the bone may also be fractured. Time is of the essence for the successful reimplantation of an avulsed permanent tooth. The tooth must be placed in a suitable storage medium within 20 minutes of its avulsion. Milk, 0.9% sodium chloride, or Hank's Balanced Salt Solution (HBSS) are good physiologic media; tap water and saliva are not. If neither milk nor 0.9% sodium chloride (contact lens solution) is available, you may be able to find HBSS in a pharmacy, either a generic brand or under the name Sav-A-Tooth® from 3M. Gently rinse the tooth with the storage medium to remove any loose dirt; do not scrape the root surface. Then submerge the tooth in the medium and head to the nearest dentist.

Successful reimplantation of the tooth depends on how long it has been out of the mouth and what the condition is of the alveolar bone from which it came. In a best case scenario, the tooth is placed in a storage medium immediately and the dentist practices next door. The alveolar bone is intact, and, after appropriate anesthesia and removal of any blood clot, the tooth is reimplanted. To ensure stability, the tooth is splinted to the teeth on either side. This splint will remain in place for approximately 1–2 weeks. Excessive splinting time leads to further complications. Antibiotics should also be administered to prevent any acute infection. A root canal will also need to be completed on the injured tooth.

The major complication after a tooth has been replanted is external root resorption. Due to the damage that the root has sustained, the body will start to resorb the root and place new bone where the root once was. There is no treatment for external root resorption. This process may continue over several years before the reimplanted tooth will have to be extracted. Reimplantation may also not be successful if the alveolar bone or the tooth root have been fractured. Generally speaking, avulsed primary teeth are not reimplanted.

Trauma to the mouth may result in a fracture of the crown of the tooth. The dentist should make sure that the tooth fragment is not embedded in the patient's lip! A favorable fracture, one which does not involve the pulp, can be repaired with a tooth-colored composite resin filling material. An unfavorable fracture will require root canal therapy and possibly a crown in order to save the tooth. The prognosis of a root fracture depends on where the fracture is located. The closer the fracture is to the apex (tip) of the root, the more favorable it is. Especially in the case of fractured anterior teeth, if one tooth is lost it may be replaced with a conventional fixed bridge or a single-tooth implant.

## WISDOM TEETH

Third molars, or wisdom teeth, have been the bane of existence for many teenagers and young adults. As humans have evolved, they have had less room in the jawbones to accommodate these teeth. In many instances these teeth are impacted, tilted against the adjacent tooth or stuck in the bone so that they cannot erupt. In other instances, the teeth erupt part way and cause problems for the adjacent tooth. The gingiva covering the wisdom tooth can become painfully infected. Thus, indications for the removal of third molars include the occurrence of pericoronitis (infected gingiva), prevention of caries on adjacent teeth or of jaw cysts and tumors or jaw fractures, orthodontic reasons, and root resorption on adjacent teeth.

The extraction procedure of third molars can range from simple to complex. If the molar is completely erupted and visible in the mouth, its removal is no more complicated than the extraction of any other multirooted tooth. If the tooth is partially or fully covered by gingiva or bone, these tissues will have to be removed first. Postoperative care is critical if discomfort is to be minimized. Proper use of analgesics, use of ice and perhaps corticosteroids to keep swelling down, refraining from smoking, and leaving the blood clot in the socket undisturbed are all contributions to an uneventful postoperative period.

## PERIORAL AND INTRAORAL ULCERS AND DERMATOLOGIC DISEASES

At one time or another, everyone has experienced an intraoral ulcer of some type. An ulcer is simply an area of tissue which has lost its epithelial covering. The ulcer is painful because the nerve endings in the connective tissue have been exposed. The area may also be inflamed.

Ulcers have a variety of causes. A traumatic ulcer occurs upon a severe bite to the cheek. This area may be repeatedly traumatized until the person subconsciously learns to avoid biting this area. Ulcers may also be caused by viruses. The most common ulcers of viral origin are those associated with the herpes virus. The six herpes-type viruses in humans are herpes simplex 1 and 2, varicella zoster, cytomegalovirus, Epstein-Barr virus, and human herpes virus 6. Herpes simplex 1 and 2 are those most commonly associated with oral lesions. Herpes virus ulcers are also referred to as cold sores or fever blisters. One major characteristic of all of the herpes viruses is that their DNA, or genetic material, can live within nerve cells. Under the appropriate conditions, either after trauma or when the host immune system is weakened, this DNA will become activated and cause the lesions. The herpetic ulcers can shed virus and infect other individuals. Any part of the body can be infected with the herpes virus. Refrain from sexual activity when you have wet, weeping viral ulcers. Do not be surprised if your dentist asks you to reschedule your appointment if you show up with a fever blister; a herpes infection can be contracted in the fingers even while one is wearing gloves!

Aphthous ulcers or canker sores are the other major type of intraoral ulcer. Aphthous ulcers have no discernible cause, although they may be stress related or have some autoimmune basis. Recurrent aphthous ulcers can be quite painful, making eating difficult. Aphthae are distinguished from herpes lesions by their location. Aphthous ulcers are seen only on moveable tissue, alveolar and buccal mucosa, within the mouth. Herpetic ulcers may be seen on the lips, moveable tissue, and gingiva.

Intraoral ulcers are often treated symptomatically. Topical anesthetics are effective at relieving pain so that the patient may eat. Severe viral ulcers may be treated with antiviral ointments or systemic medication. Viral disorders are never treated with steroids, either topical or systemic. Traumatic ulcers and aphthous ulcers heal with the tincture of time, 7–10 days if anesthetic ointments are used, 1–1½ weeks if not.

One other type of ulcerative condition is called acute necrotizing ulcerative gingivitis (ANUG). ANUG is characterized by ulceration of the tips of the gingival papillae, painful, bleeding gums, and severe bad breath. ANUG usually occurs in young individuals under stress who have poor dietary habits and insufficient oral hygiene, who smoke, and who are fatigued. It was called "trench mouth" during World War I because of the large numbers of soldiers in the trenches of France who were afflicted with the disease. ANUG is not contagious and is easily treated with a thorough cleaning of the teeth and gums, and possibly with antibiotics. A form of ANUG has been associated with a small percentage of patients who have acquired immune deficiency syndrome.

Dermatologic disorders may also manifest themselves in the mouth. Most of these disorders have an autoimmune component, meaning that the body is making antibodies and mounting an immune response against itself. Intraorally, these diseases may have as symptoms ulcerations, sloughing of the gingiva, pain, or a white, lattice-like lesion. It is important to distinguish among these diseases—lichen planus, pemphigus vulgaris, cicatricial pemphigoid, and erythema multiforme—because pemphigus may be fatal, pemphigoid may have associated ophthalmological problems, lichen planus may be precancerous (according to some researchers), and erythema multiforme may have a variety of other complications. Most of the dermatologic disorders are treated, or at least controlled, with topical and systemic steroids; more advanced cases may require simultaneous treatment by a dentist and a physician.

## ORAL CANCERS

Oral cancer is one of the 10 leading causes of death worldwide and is responsible for over 30,000 new cases of cancer in the United States each year. The major form of oral cancer is squamous cell carcinoma; it affects the epithelium which lines the mouth. The epithelial cells become malignant and virtually take over the body, eventually causing death.

Tobacco use and alcohol use, especially in combination, are cited as the major risk factors for the development of oral cancers in people in this country. Tobacco, both in the smoked and smokeless forms, accounts for significant changes in the characteristics of the oral soft tissues. Other substances such as betel nuts contribute to the high incidence of oral cancers in other countries.

Early diagnosis is beneficial in that many small tumors can be successfully removed without recurrence. For the early detection of potentially life-threatening tumors, it is imperative that prompt attention be paid to any sores or lip cracks which do not heal, lumps or bumps, color or shape changes or new hair sprouts in moles, lesions on the skin, any other lesion which does not heal or go away within 2 weeks, or lymph nodes which feel hard and do not move when pushed.

Oral cancers are treated primarily with surgical removal, radiation therapy, or both. Chemotherapy is currently only an adjunctive modality in the treatment of oral cancers. For small lesions which are detected early, surgical excision may be the only treatment needed. Patients who need radiation treatment to the head and neck area should be aware of several dental changes. If any salivary glands are in the path of the radiation beam, their ability to produce saliva will be impaired. This decrease in saliva production will result in dry-mouth syndrome. Patients with a dry mouth will be susceptible to increased and more rapid decay formation. Radiation patients should have their dental needs addressed before the commencement of the radiation therapy. This often puts the dentist at odds with the oncologist, who would like to get started immediately. If nothing else, all extractions should be completed before the initiation of the radiation therapy.

## ORAL MANIFESTATIONS OF HIV/AIDS

The epidemic of acquired immunodeficiency syndrome, or AIDS, has been a major setback to the public's health throughout the world. Recent advances in the treatment of HIV infection have given these patients new hope for an extended, productive life span. However, there is still no cure for HIV and the number of cases continues to increase.

In a small percentage of undiagnosed and diagnosed patients, oral findings are the only indication that the patient is HIV-positive. Unusual or unexplained intraoral *Candida* infections must raise suspicion about HIV status. *Candida* is an opportunistic yeast-like fungal infection and will overgrow in areas of local environmental or microbiological change. *Candida* infections are sometimes seen under poorly maintained dentures or may erupt when antibiotic therapy decreases the numbers and kinds of bacteria which usually inhabit the mouth. Impairment to the immune system such as is seen in HIV infection can also allow the *Candida* to overgrow.

In the early days of the HIV epidemic, clinicians who worked with gay populations in San Francisco and New York saw a rapid and severely destructive type of periodontitis in some of their patients. It was thought that many HIV-positive patients would have this type of disease. However, additional data indicate that it was the periodontitis that brought these patients in for care in the first place, resulting in what initially appeared to be a high rate of incidence. Recent studies suggest that severe periodontitis is seen in only a small percentage of HIV patients.

Another intraoral lesion associated with HIV is Kaposi's sarcoma. This is the most common tumor associated with HIV and is a diagnostic sign of full-blown AIDS. The lesions appear as dark red, irregularly shaped flat lesions. They are usually located on the roof of the mouth but can be on other parts of the body as well, and are sometimes surgically removed if they are unsightly. Hairy leukoplakia is a whitish lesion found on the lateral border of the tongue. While the diagnosis can only be ascertained by biopsy, the appearance of this lesion usually indicates that the HIV infection is developing into AIDS.

HIV-positive patients can receive routine dental treatment, depending on their immune status. Testing for other HIV-associated diseases such as tuberculosis and hepatitis-B is indicated. Particular attention to oral hygiene is a must, in order to keep periodontal inflammation at a minimum. Careful identification and rapid treatment of any AIDS-related disorders will keep them from further complicating already complex therapy. Patients cannot be denied treatment based solely on their HIV status. In advanced cases, however, it is prudent to seek help from a practitioner who is experienced in dealing with the myriad ramifications of this disease.

# HALITOSIS

For generations, Listerine has killed the germs that cause bad breath. A burst of Scope gets rid of "morning breath." There are endless claims from advertisers along these lines; hundreds of millions of dollars are spent annually in the search for fresher breath. So how did your breath get to smell bad in the first place? What causes the smell and what can you do to get rid of it?

Most bad breath, or halitosis, is caused by volatile sulfur compounds found in your mouth. These compounds are the result of anaerobic bacterial action and putrefaction of food debris, the natural shedding of intraoral tissues, and destruction of gingival tissues caused by periodontal disease. These bacteria also live in the crevices of the tongue. This sulfur production is exacerbated by the decrease in salivary flow while a person is sleeping. The pH of the mouth, which is usually slightly acidic, is altered by the reduced nocturnal salivary flow. Certain foods, such as onions and garlic, contribute somewhat to halitosis, as does smoking, and poorly maintained dentures can also play a part.

You can tell for yourself if you have bad breath. Take a piece of unflavored floss and clean between some of your molars. Remove the floss, wait a minute, and then smell it. If it smells bad to you, it probably does to someone else. You can check your tongue by wiping the back of it with a piece of clean gauze, waiting, and then sniffing. If you have flunked these tests, read on before grabbing for the mouthwash.

The first step in reducing halitosis is to clean your mouth completely, including in between the teeth. Plaque and food debris will collect in any nook and cranny possible. Using a brush and floss to remove both plaque and debris from all tooth surfaces is a must. Some clinicians also advocate the use of a tongue scraper. When scraped along the surface of the tongue, this simple device will remove many of the bacteria which reside in the papillae there (the tongue may also be cleaned with a toothbrush).

Recent research has suggested that rinses containing chlorine dioxide are more effective against halitosis in the long term than are the more popular brands. Chlorine dioxide acts by breaking the chemical bonds which constitute sulfur compounds. Unlike most other mouthwashes, chlorine dioxide preparations do not contain any alcohol. These chlorine dioxide-containing mouth rinses and toothpastes should be used twice daily as a normal part of the hygiene routine.

## TMJ: SYNDROME OF THE '90S

Many Americans lead high-stress, helter-skelter lives. Evidence of this stress comes in many forms, from behavior such as yelling at the kids to the presence of stomach ulcers to the use of alcohol and drugs. Clenching and grinding of the teeth is another manifestation. While there is still much to be learned in this area, there is no doubt that stress can affect the teeth, the muscles of mastication, temporomandibular joint (TMJ), and various other muscles of the neck and back.

Many people state that they "have TMJ." Technically, we all do—one temporomandibular joint on each side of the head, just in front of the ear. What these people really have is TMD, temporomandibular dysfunction. This dysfunction has many forms; there may be pain or tenderness in the teeth or in the muscles of mastication and neck muscles, or a problem with the joint itself. There is still considerable professional disagreement about what TMD is, how to diagnose it, and how to treat it. If you think you have problems with TMD, tell your dentist. Certain examination procedures not part of the routine dental exam will be performed.

It is important to remember that, as we learned in childhood, "the head bone's connected to the neck bone, the neck bone's connected to the shoulder bone" and so forth. The teeth, muscles of mastication, TMJ, and muscles of the neck and upper back are all connected to each other, either directly or by influence of other structures. Let us start with the occlusion, the way in which the teeth come together when the mouth is closed. The teeth fit together by interdigitating the hills and valleys of the posterior teeth in one jaw with the valleys and hills of the teeth in the opposite jaw. Although the teeth are designed to fit together snugly, they may not, due to the position or shape of particular teeth. Many people with malpositioned teeth have no symptoms. There is some evidence showing that malpositioned teeth may be one of the contributing factors to the occurrence of TMD. Your mandible can find the spots which do not fit together properly, and these areas can trigger clenching and/or grinding.

Clenching and grinding can have several results. Over time, teeth can be worn down or loosened in their alveolar housing. As clenching and grinding require contraction of some of the muscles of mastication, and these muscles must act against friction, there is the possibility that muscle spasms or cramps will develop. These spasms may be felt as small knots within the muscles of the face. They cause pain and may be quite sensitive when touched. Muscle spasms in the bellies of the temporalis muscle are responsible for pain on the side of the head. Spasms in the masseter and internal pterygoid muscles can account for discomfort in the cheeks. Problems with the lateral pterygoid muscle can cause discomfort by the ear. Shoulders held tightly will create spasms in the sternocleidomastoid and trapezius muscles. Pain associated with the eyes, nose, forehead, or top of the head is probably not related to TMD.

There may also be problems with the temporomandibular joint itself. The jaw is basically structured so that the tip of the mandible or the head of the condyle sits in a depression on either side of the skull. A disk-shaped piece of cartilage sits between these two bones to provide cushioning and ease of movement. The assembly is held together by several ligaments. Some of the muscles of mastication also attach in this area. Clicking or popping of the jaws may be related to the movement of the condyle against the opposing articular eminence. Noise may also emanate if the disk is not moving in complete coordination with the condyle. Clicking or popping without accompanying pain may just be an annoyance. Any pain on movement should be investigated further. Over time, or due to arthritis or trauma, a grating or grinding sound may become evident. This crepitus may signal that the structure of the joint or disk is deteriorating.

Treatment for temporomandibular dysfunction depends on the presenting symptoms and source(s) of pain. Fortunately, most TMD is occlusion/muscle related and may be treated in a straightforward fashion. If the teeth are not occluding properly, an occlusal equilibration (occlusal adjustment) may be done to reshape the teeth slightly to allow for a better fit. For those who grind, especially at night, an acrylic occlusal bite splint (bite guard, night guard) can be made. This splint is worn, usually over the upper teeth, when one goes to bed. The grinding will continue but will be against the hard, smooth surface of the splint instead of against other teeth, reducing the tension on the muscles of mastication and relieving pain. Muscle relaxers, massage, injection into the muscle spasm itself, and warm compresses are also used to treat muscle-related TMD. If the TMJ itself is deteriorating, some practitioners recommend surgery of the joint, although this is becoming more controversial. In the worst cases, little can be done to completely eliminate the discomfort.

# 7. Your High-Tech Dentist

Dentists, by their very nature, love gadgets, and there is enough low- and high-tech equipment to keep even the most demanding ones satisfied. Over the past 15 years, technological advances have improved the quality of your dental care.

You are probably familiar with the ultrasonic unit your dentist or hygienist uses to clean your teeth. Since its introduction in the 1950s, this powered cleaning unit has become more effective. It can also deliver a variety of liquid medications and use a fine jet of sodium bicarbonate to clean the stain from your teeth. When you need a composite resin restoration, the resin is polymerized by a curing unit which emits a bright light. This light activates the catalyst in the plastic, and the resin polymerizes.

Most patients find getting the shot of anesthetic to be the least palatable part of their dental appointment. Hand-held transcutaneous electrical nerve stimulation (TENS) units are available that allow you to control how numb your tissues are. The anesthesia provided by TENS is enough for a comfortable teeth-cleaning and even for the placing of some restorations. If nothing else, you can use it to numb yourself while you are receiving your injection of local anesthetic for more extensive procedures. Unfortunately, TENS units do not work on everyone. If your dentist has one, you will need to experiment with it to find the proper setting; one that is too low is ineffective, and one that is too high can make the TENS effect uncomfortable in itself.

Many dental offices are now computerized for most business operations. Billing, scheduling, insurance filing, and many other accounting functions are automated in the modern practice. The computer has also found its way into diagnostic equipment and into the fabrication of some restorations. As we will see in chapter 8, subtraction radiography uses a computer to subtract one X-ray film image from another of the same area. The advantage of this is to make the films much more sensitive to changes in tooth structure or bone. Instead of needing a 30% change in density before detection is possible, subtraction radiographs are sensitive down to 5%. Computer assisted design/computer assisted manufacture (CAD/CAM) has entered the world of dental restorations. Metal or porcelain restorations may be created with one of these machines, which uses lasers to map the surface of the tooth. Through the use of sophisticated computer programming, a piece of gold or porcelain can then be milled to fit the exact shape of the prepared tooth. At present, this is still costly technology, so only a few dentists and dental schools have the necessary equipment.

Computers also serve as the backbone for the new imaging systems. An intraoral camera can be used to make pictures of the existing conditions in your mouth. These images may then be stored on disks or printed out as a hard record. Being able to see clearly, on a computer screen, what the problems are helps you better understand what is going on in your mouth. Producing instantaneous pictures also enables your dentist to send these to your insurance company to support a claim for treatment. Cosmetic dentists, oral surgeons, and plastic surgeons can use these images in conjunction with modification software to change your appearance on the video screen. You are able to obtain a reasonably (not perfectly) accurate assessment of your new look after undergoing cosmetic dentistry procedures.

Lasers have received a lot of attention over the past five years. In many instances, the laser is a piece of hot technology looking for a home in dentistry. It plays a role, albeit a small one, in periodontics and oral surgery, being, in effect, a very expensive scalpel. One major advantage is that the laser minimizes bleeding at the surgical site; another is that its use may result in less postoperative discomfort for the patient than in conventional surgery. Carbon dioxide lasers are used most often for soft tissue surgery. Nd:Yag and other lasers have been used to prepare teeth for restorations. The laser has been touted as a tool that will eliminate the need for drills and anesthetic, but this is not entirely accurate. While progress has been made, the laser has its drawbacks and, as of now, has not been widely embraced for use in restorative dentistry.

Some low-tech items have received attention lately. More dentists are using magnification, usually in the form of loupes, as well as better lighting. Magnification greatly improves the clinician's ability to see the finer points of his or her work, whether it is looking for a piece of calculus on a root, exploring a tooth for a minute fracture, or checking the margins of a restoration for proper fit. Fiber-optic wands also assist in detecting cracks in teeth and other minor flaws. Endodontists, periodontists, and oral surgeons are increasingly turning to the use of surgical microscopes for their operations.

While technology is a tremendous helpmate, good dentistry still depends on that greatest computer of all, the human brain. Excellent practitioners can elevate their treatment to the highest levels with the latest technology. Poor clinicians will remain just that, only with fancy equipment. You should not judge your dentist's skill solely by the instruments and equipment that are found in the office.

# 8. Research Trends: Toward the Twenty-First Century

The practice of dentistry today is not what it was a generation, or even 5 years, ago. Progress is continually being made in many areas, such as practitioners' better understanding of the disease process and the development of new treatment techniques, restorative materials, instruments, and equipment. In most instances, progress is evolutionary, not revolutionary. In the past 150 years, revolutionary changes in dentistry have included the introduction of amalgam, the use of local anesthetics, the advent of the high-speed turbine drill (which happened only in the 1950s), the introduction of composite resin materials, and the recognition of bacterial plaque as the primary cause of caries and periodontal disease. Other advances can be marked against these milestones.

Predicting what the future holds is an uncertain business at best. While some areas of research have matured, it is the unexpected findings which bring excitement to the art of discovery. Following are some research trends as ascertained from the dental scientific literature.

## PREVENTION

Work on vaccines against caries and the periodontal diseases has slowed significantly. At one time it was felt that developing a vaccine against specific bacteria would offer protection against the two chronic diseases which affect more people worldwide than any other. Two problems have been encountered. First, bacteria tend to mutate so that the vaccine becomes ineffective. Second, while the group of bacteria reputed to cause periodontal disease has been identified, there is still no evidence to suggest that one or two specific bacteria are responsible for the initiation of periodontal inflammation. Hence, which bacteria should the vaccine be made against? Currently, new antimicrobial agents are being tested in toothpastes and mouth rinses in the fight against plaque. Triclosan, a type of detergent, has been used effectively in Europe for many years, and triclosan-containing products are now being test marketed in the United States. Some studies are investigating the anticaries effect of xylitol, the artificial sweetener found in some chewing gums. Xylitol may cause a decrease in caries because the *Streptococcus species* and other bacteria responsible for the decay process cannot metabolize it; additional protection comes from the increase in salivary flow when gum is chewed. In studying sealants, composite resins have been shown to be far superior to the newer glass ionomer materials.

The anticaries benefits resulting from low levels of fluoride in drinking water (1 part per million) have been known for decades. Still, only approximately 60–70% of the public water supplies in this country contain this level of fluoride. You may want to check with your water supply company, and do something about it if the water is not fluoridated.

## DIAGNOSTICS

The trend in diagnosis involves the ability to predict what teeth or periodontal pockets are susceptible to either caries or periodontal disease. There are in-office tests to identify which caries-causing bacteria are present in the mouth. There are also tests to detect various indicators of periodontal inflammation. Two problems still need to be worked out. First, since it is impractical and expensive to test all sites, which ones should be tested? Second, will the information obtained change treatment in any way? If your dentist cannot answer this question to your satisfaction, perhaps the test should not be done. One set of tests, though, is very valuable for periodontal diseases which have not responded to conventional treatment. Obtaining a plaque sample from a pocket which continues to bleed and having these bacteria cultured and identified can give your dentist information on which antibiotic(s) to use in trying to eliminate the infection. Although, as we have seen, systemic antibiotics are not used routinely, they are definitely indicated when problems persist.

Standard dental radiographs can detect changes in tooth structure or bone only after approximately 30% of the density is lost. As noted in chapter 7, a newer technique, called subtraction radiography, can improve density detection down to a 5% change. This computer-driven technology takes two radiographs made over time and digitally subtracts one image from the other. The result is the change in density in specific areas. This technology can detect new carious lesions much earlier and measure bone loss due to periodontal disease or bone gain after regenerative periodontal surgery. While still in the experimental stage, this technology should be available to most dentists within the next 10 years.

## RESTORATIVE DENTISTRY

In spite of the often anecdotal nay-saying by a few practitioners, dental amalgam is still one of the major materials used in restorative dentistry. Recent evidence suggests that, while those patients who have amalgam fillings and dentists who place amalgam restorations have slightly higher urinary mercury concentration than others, these people do not have any more or greater health problems than those with lower mercury levels. Apparently, this debate will continue for scientific and unscientific reasons. One trend is becoming obvious: with the improvement of other dental materials, amalgam use is beginning to show a significant decrease.

Product development continues with tooth-colored restorative materials. New generations of composite resins appear regularly; while they are still more difficult to place than amalgam, as their wear properties improve they will be used more for fillings in posterior teeth. Glass ionomer restorative materials and cements also continue to improve, although these materials do not have the wear or aesthetic characteristics of composites. Significant progress has been made in the use of porcelain veneers for anterior teeth and porcelain restorations for posterior teeth. Porcelain makes the restoration almost invisible to the naked eye.

## PERIODONTICS

The most significant research involves the application of molecular biology to periodontal pathogenesis, diagnosis, and treatment. Test kits for enzymes detectable in the fluid which seeps from the gingival margin are available. Several questions remain. Which substance should be analyzed? Which sites should be checked? What does this information mean vis-à-vis treatment?

The most substantial research is being done in the realm of periodontal regeneration. The ideal dental treatment aims to restore the lost body in as natural a state as possible. While bone grafting can restore bone, and guided tissue regeneration can help create a new periodontal ligament as well, these procedures are not completely predictable and cannot be used in all cases of periodontal destruction. Current work centers on the use of growth proteins to stimulate new bone and connective tissue formation. Several substances are being tested, some derived as a result of genetic engineering. Recombinant bone morphogenetic protein 2 seems to significantly accelerate bone growth when used with other bone graft materials. Work is being done on identifying the appropriate growth factors and the correct delivery system.

## RESEARCH YOU CAN USE

New consumer dental products are continually appearing in the marketplace, including toothbrush designs, powered toothbrushes, mouth rinses, bleaching agents, toothpastes, floss, and auxiliary hygiene aids. Before running out to buy the latest product, ask yourself three questions. (1) Am I able to maintain my oral health with what I am currently using? If the answer is yes, why fool with success? The only reason to switch, besides boredom, is that the new product will make maintaining your oral health easier *without any loss in effectiveness!* Change for the sake of change, especially if you end up worse off than before, does not make sense. (2) Does the product do what the ads claim it will do? (3) Even if the product does what it claims to do (such as reduce plaque), does it have a positive effect on my oral health? You may need to consult your dentist to get some help with these questions. As much as we would all like it, there is no magic bullet for good oral health.

# 9. Where to Go for Further Information

I hope that this book has made you more knowledgeable and more curious about your own oral health. Your best source of information now is your general dentist, who can provide you with a detailed diagnosis and treatment plan for any oral problems, and who can refer you to a specialist if you have a condition which he or she does not feel comfortable treating. As I directed you in chapter 2, ask, ask, ask questions, and then ask some more. You are entitled to as much information about your mouth as you would like.

Besides being able to give you specific information, many dentists have pamphlets on a wide range of dental topics. These publications are produced by many different groups, such as the American Dental Association, various specialty groups, dental consumer product manufacturers, and other commercial companies. Many of these brochures are well illustrated and can provide you with a lot of information.

Another source of information, although it is one that should be viewed cautiously, is the newspaper. When news items highlight a recent study or publication, it is often out of context with what is going on in the rest of dentistry. While a news piece will give you some information, applying it to your particular situation without consulting your dentist can be misleading. For instance, at one time the newspapers played up the use of baking soda and peroxide for controlling periodontal disease. While the application of these items has been and sometimes still is advocated, many readers were given the false impression that this was all that was necessary to maintain good periodontal health. In reality, the use of these two substances was but one part of a complex method of treatment, microbiologically modulated periodontal therapy (MMPT), originally presented by Dr. Paul

Keyes. MMPT included thorough oral hygiene, scaling and root planing, the use of antimicrobials, antibiotics, and possibly surgery to control the disease. The "Keyes technique" has many valid points, but the press often focused on one—baking soda and peroxide—to the exclusion of the more difficult but equally necessary parts of therapy. This misled some readers into thinking that all of their problems could be solved with this magic potion.

Many articles highlighting advances in dentistry also appear in magazines, especially women's magazines. These articles usually focus on one aspect of dentistry, such as implants, aesthetics, or periodontal disease. Most are well written and give some general information. Facts presented in such places can serve as a good springboard from which to make inquiries of your dentist. In my opinion, the best articles on dental health and products appear periodically in *Consumer Reports*. These pieces, uniformly well researched, evenhanded, and accurate, may focus on the evaluation of oral health care products or may concentrate on various aspects of dental care.When controversy exists, viewpoints from all sides are presented.

Television has done a lot to heighten many people's awareness of good oral hygiene. Toothbrush, toothpaste, and mouthwash commercials have all targeted home care as an integral part of maintaining oral health. We all know that one mouthwash, which used to kill the germs that cause bad breath, now also kills the germs that cause gingivitis (and the company has good scientific studies to prove it). These advertisers want to sell you their products, so they may not tell the whole story. In addition, some so-called "news items" which you may see on the local or national news are no more than extended commercials. Manufacturers will send press releases to the ever-hungry media, hoping that their product may be featured in a report. Do not give credence to a new product just because it was in a news snippet unless it is part of a broader, more balanced report.

# Appendix A: Suggestions for Further Reading

There are many dental textbooks and some consumer-oriented books about dental health on the market today. While the texts are written for dental students and practitioners, many are appropriate for the well-educated reader. If you read one of these books, remember to keep everything in context, or you may decide that you have each disease mentioned!

## BOOKS

*A Consumer's Guide to Dentistry* by Gorden J. Christensen, D.D.S., M.S.D., Ph.D. This well-illustrated book goes into detail about many of the concepts and issues discussed in *Understanding Dental Health*. St. Louis: Mosby-Year Book, 1994.

*Change Your Smile* (3rd ed.) by Ronald E. Goldstein, D.D.S. This book presents a tremendous amount of detail on the various aesthetic dental problems and their solutions. Topics covered include bleaching, bonding, veneers, orthodontics, and orthognathic surgery. Chicago: Quintessence, 1996.

*Primary Preventive Dentistry* (4th ed.) by Norman O. Harris, D.D.S., M.S.D., and Arden G. Christen, D.D.S., M.S.D., M.A. This basic text details the mechanisms of the two most prevalent dental diseases and enumerates various preventive approaches to them. A well-referenced and complete work, it is not light reading but is very informative. Norwalk: Appleton and Lange, 1995.

## CYBERSPACE

Cyberspace is also a potential source of dental information. At last count, there were over 1500 dental sites from which to choose. Most of the major dental organizations, dental specialty organizations and academies, dental schools, and many private practices maintain home pages. The content of these home pages changes regularly and some are more valuable than others. As those of you with Internet experience know, it is possible to waste significant amounts of time wandering through cyberspace. In addition, some sites referenced have nothing to do with dentistry, and a few are quite offensive. In order to save you some time, a few of the more interesting and valuable sites are listed below (as of January 1997).

American Dental Association (ADA ONLINE)—
http://www.ada.org

The American Dental Association is the primary organization representing all dentists in the United States. The ADA maintains a service called ADA ONLINE, which has four different major components. News includes *Dental News Digest*, previews of the *ADA News* and other news items. Practice & Profession offers dental education and career information, ADA statements on a variety of issues important to the profession, and an events calendar. Products & Services features the list of products with the ADA Seal of Acceptance, information about ADA member services, and the *ADA Catalog*. Consumer Information provides information on fluoride, dental amalgam, baby-bottle tooth decay, oral hygiene, diet, endodontics, periodontics, sealants, and dental insurance benefits. In addition, at the end of the "News" component of the site is a listing of many other accessible Web sites. The accessible dental sites include those of dental associations and societies, dental schools, and other dental organizations, as well as medical sites, nondental association sites, business, cultural, entertainment, travel, science, government, and newsstand sites. A Web tools and resources directory is also included. All sites are accessible to the general public. The ADA may also be reached by phone at 1-800-621-8099.

Canadian Dental Association—
**http://cda-adc.ca/english/**
This is the major organization representing Canadian dentists.
The site maintains information and tips for the dental consumer.

Academy of General Dentistry—
**http://www.agd.org**
The AGD represents about 30,000 general dentists in the
United States. Its Website features abstracts of articles from its
journal and newsletter as well as consumer information.

California Dental Hygienists Association—
**http://www.toothfairy.org**
This is the state association for California's dental hygienists.
An interesting and entertaining site, it provides good links to
current information on periodontics.

Baylor College of Dentistry—
**http://www.ont.com/baylords**
Offering a wide range of information regarding the various
aspects of dentistry, career opportunities, and academic
programs, this site is also accessible through ADA ONLINE.

University of North Carolina—
**http://www.dent.unc.edu/careers/cidtoc.htm**
This site has an in-depth presentation on the various career
opportunities in dentistry.

# Appendix B: Dental Schools

Dental schools are a primary resource for any type of dental information. There are 54 dental schools in the United States, all of which are affiliated with major universities. You may wish to get your dental care at such a school. This would mean trading time for money; treatment will take longer, but the fees may be considerably less than in the private sector. Remember that dental students, although supervised by well-qualified faculty, are still learning their profession.

Some dental schools and many community colleges also sponsor dental hygiene programs. While it is not possible to have all of your dental needs met through these programs, the dental hygiene students can help you focus on prevention and on maintaining your periodontal health. All programs have dentists on faculty to answer your questions and help make the appropriate referral if you need further care.

Schools are listed by state or Canadian province. Information is current as of January 1997.

**Alabama**
University of Alabama at Birmingham
School of Dentistry
1919 7th Avenue South, Suite 406
Birmingham, AL 35294-0007
205-934-3000

**California**
Loma Linda University
School of Dentistry
11092 Anderson Street
Loma Linda, CA 92354
909-824-4222

University of California at Los
Angeles
School of Dentistry
Center for the Health Sciences
Los Angeles, CA 90024-1668
310-825-7354

University of California at San
Francisco
School of Dentistry
513 Parnassus Avenue, Rm. S-630
San Francisco, CA 94143-0430
415-476-1323

University of the Pacific
School of Dentistry
2155 Webster Street
San Francisco, CA 94115
415-929-6400

University of Southern California
School of Dentistry
University Park - MC-0641
Los Angeles, CA 90089-0641
213-740-2800

**Colorado**
University of Colorado
School of Dentistry
4200 E. Ninth Avenue
Box C-284
Denver, CO 80262
303-315-8752

**Connecticut**
University of Connecticut
School of Dental Medicine
263 Farmington Avenue
Farmington, CT 06030-3915
860-679-2808

**District of Columbia**
Howard University
College of Dentistry
600 W. Street, NW
Washington, DC 20059-0001
202-806-0100

**Florida**
University of Florida
College of Dentistry
1600 SW Archer Road, Room D4-6
P. O. Box 100405
Gainesville, FL 32610-0405
352-392-2946

**Georgia**
Medical College of Georgia
School of Dentistry
1120 15th Street, Rm. AD1119
Augusta, GA 30912-1000
706-721-0211

**Illinois**
Northwestern University
Dental School
240 E. Huron St.
Chicago, IL 60611-2972
312-503-6837

Southern Illinois University
School of Dental Medicine
2800 College Avenue
Alton, IL 62002-4789
618-474-7000

University of Illinois at Chicago
College of Dentistry
801 S. Paulina Street
Chicago, IL 60612-7211
312-996-7520

**Indiana**
Indiana University
School of Dentistry
1121 W. Michigan Street
Indianapolis, IN 46202-5186
317-274-7957

**Iowa**
University of Iowa
College of Dentistry
100 Dental Science Building
Iowa City, IA 52242-1010
319-335-9650

**Kentucky**
University of Kentucky
College of Dentistry
800 Rose Street
Lexington, KY 40536-0084
606-323-5850

University of Louisville
School of Dentistry
501 S. Preston
Louisville, KY 40292
502-852-5293

**Louisiana**
Louisiana State University
School of Dentistry
1100 Florida Avenue
New Orleans, LA 70119
504-619-9961

**Maryland**
University of Maryland at Baltimore
Dental School
666 W. Baltimore Street
Baltimore, MD 21201
410-706-7460

**Massachusetts**
Boston University
Goldman School of Dental Medicine
100 E. Newton Street
Boston, MA 02118
617-638-4700

Harvard School of Dental Medicine
188 Longwood Avenue
Boston, MA 02115
617-432-1405

Tufts University
School of Dental Medicine
1 Kneeland Street
Boston, MA 02111
617-636-7000

**Michigan**
University of Detroit Mercy
School of Dentistry
2985 E. Jefferson Avenue
Detroit, MI 48207-4282
313-446-1800

University of Michigan
School of Dentistry
1011 North University Avenue
Ann Arbor, MI 48109-1078
313-763-6933

**Minnesota**
University of Minnesota
School of Dentistry
515 Delaware Street SE
15-209 Moos Tower
Minneapolis, MN 55455
612-625-9982

**Mississippi**
University of Mississippi
School of Dentistry
2500 N. State Street
Jackson, MS 39216-4505
601-984-6000

**Missouri**
University of Missouri-Kansas City
School of Dentistry
650 E. 25th Street
Kansas City, MO 64108-2784
816-235-2100

**Nebraska**
Creighton University
School of Dentistry
2500 California Plaza
Omaha, NE 68178-0240
402-280-5060

University of Nebraska Medical
    Center
College of Dentistry
40th and Holdrege Streets
Lincoln, NE 68583-0740
402-472-1301

**New Jersey**
University of Medicine and Dentistry
    of New Jersey
New Jersey Dental School
110 Bergen Street
Newark, NJ 07103-2400
201-982-4300

**New York**
Columbia University
School of Dental and Oral Surgery
630 W. 168th Street
New York, NY 10032
212-305-2500

New York University
College of Dentistry
345 East 24th Street
New York, NY 10010-4099
212-998-9800

State University of New York at
    Buffalo
School of Dental Medicine
325 Squire Hall, 3435 Main Street
Buffalo, NY 14214-3008
716-829-2821